This book is dedicated to every woman in the world who has ever had a bad hair day, a bad man day…or a bad life day!

It's for the woman sitting on the sofa in her tracksuit bottoms, feeling like her best days are behind her, and the woman who is suddenly motivated to find a better future.

And it's also for my little daughter, Ciara, who I hope knows that when she's all grown up and maybe a mum like me, that no matter what her shape and size, she is lovely and special in every way.

COLEEN NOLAN'S

Beauty Secrets

The real woman's guide to looking gorgeous,
whatever your age, shape or size

SIDGWICK & JACKSON

First published 2010 by Sidgwick & Jackson
an imprint of Pan Macmillan, a division of Macmillan Publishers Limited
Pan Macmillan, 20 New Wharf Road, London N1 9RR
Basingstoke and Oxford
Associated companies throughout the world
www.panmacmillan.com

ISBN 978-0-283-07112-6 HB

1 3 5 7 9 8 6 4 2

A CIP catalogue record for this book is available from
the British Library.

Art Directed and Designed by Nikki Dupin/www.nicandlou.com
Photography © Nicky Johnston
Illustrations © Veronica Palmieri

Additional photographic sources:
Benoît Audureau: 52, 53, 55, 58, 59
REX FEATURES: Universal Pictures UK 9, Mark Campbell 15. Ken Mckay/ITV/157
GETTY IMAGES: Sony Music Archive/Getty Images 9, Creative Crop 37, Peter Cade 41, Andrew McCaul 50,
Turqueti 56, Image Source 57, David De Stefano 62, BBS United 63, Image Source 70, Jennifer Cheung 75,
Charles Nesbit 88, Nicki Dowey 104, Ronnie Kaufman 118, Mike Kemp 120, Tetra Images 125,
Gavin Kingcome Photography 128, Brian Klutch 138, Stockbyte 191, Michael Rosenfeld, 219.

Printed and bound in Italy by Rotolito

Visit **www.panmacmillan.com** to read more about all our books and to buy them. You will also find features,
author interviews and news of any author events, and you can sign up for e-newsletters so that you're always
first to hear about our new releases.

CONTENTS

INTRODUCTION   *I'm in the mood*   6

CHAPTER 1   *Attention to me*
Discovering What You've Got to Work With   12

CHAPTER 2   *Don't it make my brown eyes blue*
Your Face and Make-up   28

CHAPTER 3   *Spirit, body and soul*
Your Body   66

CHAPTER 4   *Don't make waves*
Your Hair   90

CHAPTER 5   *Touch me in the morning*
Your Hands and Feet   122

CHAPTER 6   *Let's get physical*
Exercise and Diet   144

CHAPTER 7   *Gotta pull myself together*
Looking Your Best   172

CHAPTER 8   *I will survive*
Feeling Good Inside   200

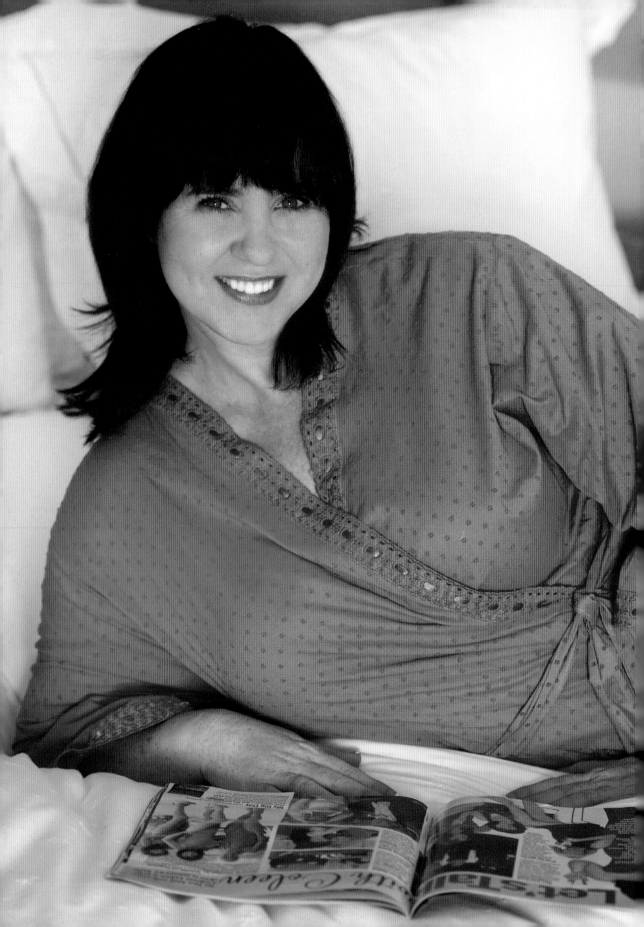

I'm in the mood...

INTRODUCTION

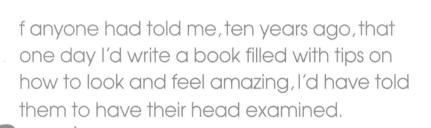

*I*f anyone had told me, ten years ago, that one day I'd write a book filled with tips on how to look and feel amazing, I'd have told them to have their head examined.

It all started out well. At fifteen, when I was singing with my sisters in The Nolans, my skin had that fresh bloom of youth and I had the enviable figure of a teenager. Travelling the world and having fabulous wardrobes to choose from gave me masses of confidence and self-esteem.

For years I took pride in my appearance and picked up the tricks and tips of the best beauty experts and make-up artists, who were paid to transform us into glittering pop stars. With no children to run around after and a demanding, successful job that I loved, I could look in the mirror and not feel too unhappy with the girl smiling back at me.

But then it all went horribly wrong. I gave up the career I'd worked so hard for and found myself in an unhappy marriage that sapped my confidence. Every day was filled with looking after the children and, once the boys were in bed, I'd spend hours alone as my then husband, Shane Ritchie, worked away from home. I could go days without seeing anyone other than the kids, and before I knew it I was slobbing about the house in tracksuit bottoms, overweight and desperately miserable.

I was an unfit, unhealthy woman who looked and felt like her best years were behind her. And yet here I am, having the time of my life, writing a book that I hope will make you feel as wonderful as I do now.

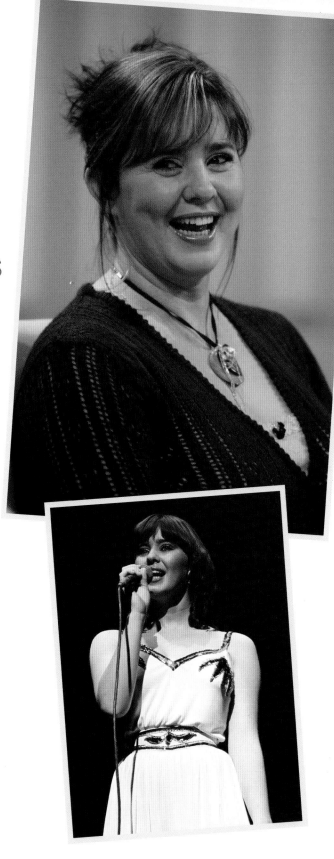

'I WAS AN UNFIT, UNHEALTHY WOMAN WHO LOOKED AND FELT LIKE HER BEST YEARS WERE BEHIND HER'

Don't get me wrong. I'm no picture of perfection. I have my lumps and bumps and bits I'd rather keep covered up, thank you very much. And I still have to reach for my make-up bag if I don't want to scare the horses.

I don't have the time or the desire to spend hours pampering myself. As a busy working mum of three I wouldn't want to use precious hours that could be spent with the family obsessing about cellulite or laughter lines.

And, having worked hard for every penny I've got, I can't be doing with wasting money on the latest too-good-to-be-true wonder products. Who can justify splashing out £100 on a pot of face cream? My mum never spent a shilling on herself and I don't remember her having a wrinkle – not even in her eighties!

So the new me has not come about because I suddenly found ten extra hours in the day to primp and pamper myself, or because I spent squillions finding the secret of eternal youth. No, this new me is one I've uncovered by working hard to make some changes, remembering the Coleen I used to be and finding the self-confidence to take care of her.

For me, making the change meant losing 5 stone. And having lost the weight – through eating sensibly and finding a type of exercise I actually enjoy – I wanted to take pride in my hair, my skin, my hands and my feet, and rediscover the joys of clothes and make-up.

I admit that after that original weight loss, a few pounds crept back on. But my weight has stabilised and now I can finally look in the mirror and, on a good day and with a fair wind, once again see the youngest Nolan smiling back. And do you know what? It's great.

So, that's the good news. I'm proof that it's never too late to make changes and that by following a few simple rules and using clever beauty tricks, you too can look in the mirror and like what you see.

The tougher news is that you can't just sit around in those old tracksuit bottoms and expect to look amazing without making a bit of an effort. I know what it's like. When you're tired after a long day looking after the kids or doing your best at work, the last thing you feel like is some dry-skin brushing, a complicated face pack and squeezing yourself into something slinky and a pair of high heels. It's all a bit too much like hard work.

And even if you can be bothered, these days we all want instant results, despite the fact that we can't all afford to pay for them. Cosmetic surgery has never been more in demand, with women (and men) searching for the secret of eternal youth.

I believe happiness lies somewhere in between all of the above. If you look younger, you will feel happier. But anti-ageing doesn't have to involve a trip to the plastic surgeon. We're meant to have laughter lines and individual noses – what a terrible world it would be if we all looked the same (although if I looked a little more like Angelina Jolie I could live with it). But on a more serious note, I know I would never be happy looking in the mirror if I'd been under the surgeon's knife.

'I'VE GONE FROM BEING UNFIT AND MISERABLE TO BEING HAPPIER THAN I'VE EVER FELT IN MY LIFE'

By combining some old-fashioned family secrets with clever expert tips I've collected along the way, I now have my own bag of tricks that I'm dying to share with you. They include ideas on how to keep your face radiant, your hair shiny, your eyes bright and your skin in top condition. They won't take up hours of your valuable time and they won't cost you the earth.

I also want to pass on what I've learned over the years about how to dress for your shape (whatever it is), how to work wonders fast with some crafty make-up tips and how eating and drinking healthily doesn't have to involve jojoba beans and weird macrobiotic salads.

There's a section on easy exercises that will boost your energy levels and improve your health. If you saw me skating on *Dancing on Ice*, you'll know we're not talking Madonna levels of fitness and flexibility here, so don't panic! I'm proof that it's possible to have fun and get fit at the same time.

I'll be looking at how stress can sap your confidence, make you head for the biscuit tin and take its toll on your appearance. But most importantly I hope this book will encourage you to rediscover yourself. To forget the excuses we all make and to realise that looking great and feeling amazing is possible for each and every one of us. Beauty is not just for the rich and famous, the posh and pampered. Real beauty is within real women and can be found by those with the smallest of incomes and the busiest of lives.

So, put away those tracksuit bottoms, go easy on the pizza and chocolate biscuits (just for now; they'll still be there when you need the occasional treat) and celebrate who you really are. We'll take it very gently and you'll soon ditch those old excuses.

I've gone from being unfit and miserable to being happier than I've ever felt in my life. And if I can do it, you can too…

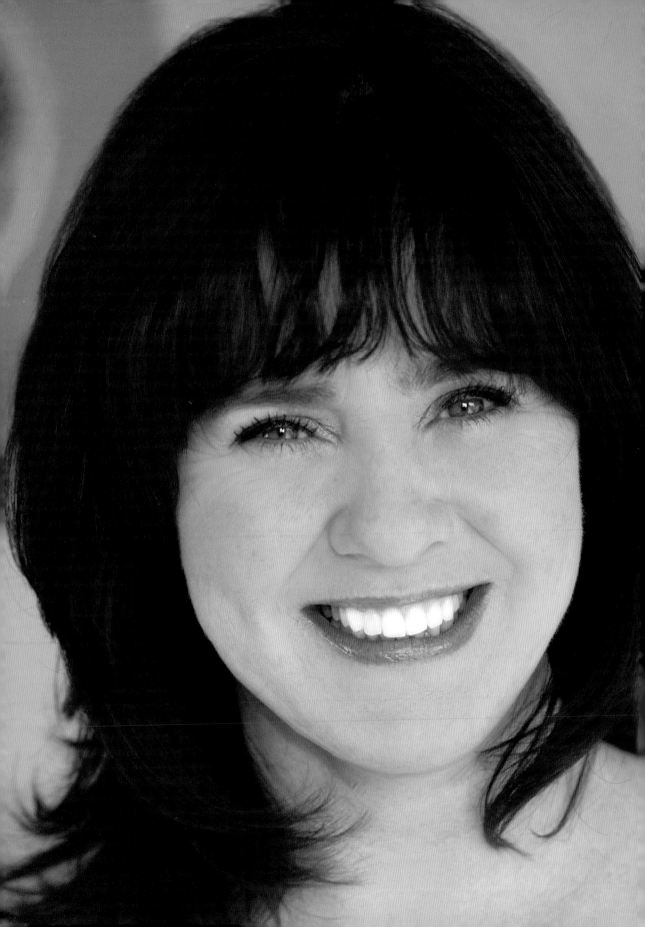

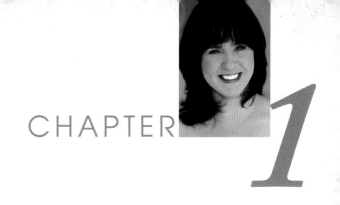

CHAPTER 1

Attention to me...

DISCOVERING WHAT YOU'VE GOT TO WORK WITH

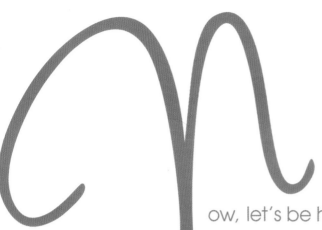

ow, let's be honest with each other. The very fact that you've bought this book makes me think there are bits of your body (or your life) that you're unhappy with. Am I right? My God, yes! I hear you say. Unless you have the face of Cheryl Cole, the hair of Jennifer Aniston and the figure of a *Strictly Come Dancing* professional, there's always room for improvement.

But before we begin to take steps towards the new you, we have to take a long, hard look at the current model. **WARNING:** this involves the removal of some clothing and extreme close-ups in harsh lighting, but try to be brave.

I realised recently why I'm finally so happy. It's because I don't try too hard to please others. As I've got older I've learned to accept myself for what I am and I don't pretend to be anything more or less. I'm a mother of three, in her forties, who will never again know the pleasure of fitting into a size-8 dress, but who really doesn't mind (much).

Going back on tour with my sisters was amazing because we did it as middle-aged women, not mutton-dressed-as-lamb wannabes. It was fantastic, and our male fans didn't seem to mind much either!

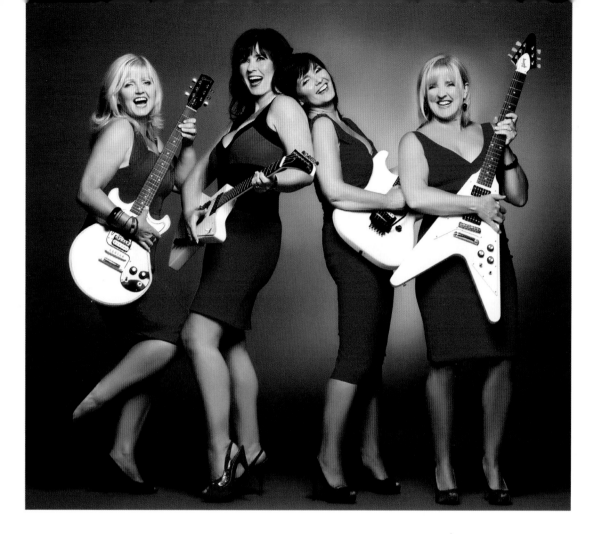

'GOING BACK ON TOUR WITH MY SISTERS WAS AMAZING BECAUSE WE DID IT AS MIDDLE-AGED WOMEN. IT WAS FANTASTIC'

We all agreed that the reason we felt so good was because after so many years we finally knew what suited us. We knew our body shapes and we knew how to avoid the disasters of the past. In other words, we recognised the raw materials and we knew what we had to work with.

Now it's time for you to do the same. Follow my instructions on how to analyse your face, body, hair, fitness and stress levels, and then later on in the book we'll use that knowledge in the pursuit of gorgeousness.

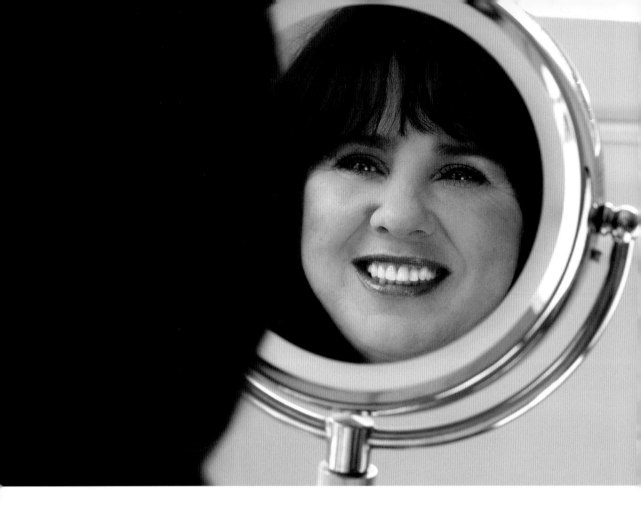

FACE

WHEN WAS THE LAST TIME YOU REALLY LOOKED AT YOUR FACE? AT ITS SHAPE, ITS SKIN TYPE AND COLOUR, AND ITS COMPLEXION?

- Begin by finding a large, clear mirror. Move it to natural light near a window.

- Using a hairband, sweep your hair off your face and remove every last scrap of make-up; do not tone or moisturise.

- Leave your skin to settle for a short while before giving it a really close examination.

What Is Your Skin Type?

Normal Skin

Lucky you! If you can cleanse your face without it feeling as tight as a drum twenty minutes later, or go through the day without worrying that you have oil slicks around your forehead, nose and chin, then you've been blessed with normal skin. You have clear skin that isn't sensitive or prone to breaking out in spots. You still have to follow a daily cleansing and moisturising regime, but if you do, you should escape the curse of zits and dry patches.

Oily Skin

A mixed blessing. Oily skin, especially around the forehead, nose and chin, will give you a shiny, greasy complexion that can lead to spots and blackheads. You'll know if this is your skin type because your skin will never feel really clean and fresh apart from immediately after cleansing. But the good news is the excess oil will help your skin look younger for longer.

Dry Skin

Does your face sometimes feel tight and your skin look thin or stretched? And do you see broken veins under the surface? Your dry complexion means the lack of protective oils will leave your skin prone to lines, so make sure you moisturise.

Sensitive Skin

You won't need me to tell you if you have sensitive skin. Cleansers, moisturisers and cosmetics that aren't hypo-allergenic will irritate your face and leave it burning or feeling itchy. Certain foods may also cause a reaction, leading to blotchy or bumpy skin or dryness.

Combination Skin

You may have a mixture of dry and oily skin – drier on the cheeks and greasier in the central zone around the forehead, nose and chin. You don't have to be a rocket scientist to realise that you will need to treat these areas differently, but don't fork out on lots of different products; just address the area that troubles you most and use a little common sense.

What Is Your Face Shape?

There are **five basic face shapes**, and knowing your face shape is important, both when applying make-up and choosing the perfect hairstyle. Look carefully at the bone structure of your face, at your cheekbones and cheeks, your forehead and the line of your jaw.

Read each of the descriptions carefully before deciding which suits your own face shape.

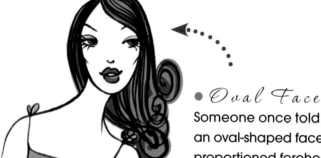

• *Oval Face*

Someone once told me that almost all top models have an oval-shaped face. With high cheekbones, a well-proportioned forehead and jaw line and a delicate chin, most hairstyles will look amazing. So if this is you, enjoy!

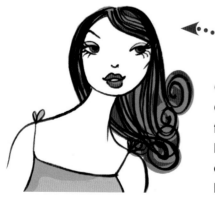

• *Round Face*

Can you draw an imaginary circle starting at your forehead, round the left cheek, chin, right cheek and back up to the forehead? If so, you have a round face and there are certain haircuts that should be avoided. More of this later in the book.

'KNOWING YOUR FACE SHAPE IS IMPORTANT WHEN APPLYING MAKE-UP AND CHOOSING THE PERFECT HAIRSTYLE'

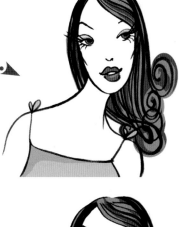

● *Square Face*

A wide forehead, hard-to-find cheekbones and a strong, square jaw line? Your square-shaped face can be striking and attractive, but you may need a more feminine haircut to soften your features. I'll describe the best haircuts for your face shape later in the book.

● *Long Face*

Do you have a high forehead? Or a long chin? Or both? These features will give your face a longish appearance and you'll want to avoid very short or very long hairstyles that will exaggerate this.

● *Heart-Shaped Face*

You have a wider forehead, high cheekbones and a cute, pointy chin. Find out how to make the most of your face shape later on.

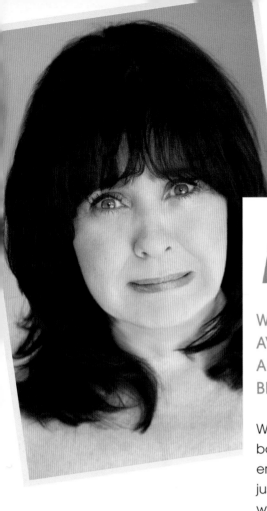

BODY

WHEN I WAS AT MY HEAVIEST I COVERED UP AND AVOIDED MIRRORS. I UNDRESSED IN THE DARK AND COULDN'T HAVE TOLD YOU WHAT MY BEST BITS WERE – I DIDN'T THINK I HAD ANY!

What I'd forgotten is that by knowing more about my body shape I could have camouflaged the bad and emphasised the good. I could have flattered my figure just by knowing what clothing styles suited me best. Losing weight doesn't change anything: your basic structure will remain the same.

OK, NOW FOR THE BRAVE BIT:

- Choose a time when you know you aren't going to be interrupted by the kids, your partner, the dog or the milkman (you never know!).

- Find a full-length mirror and, if you can bear it, take off all your clothes. You can strip down to your undies if you'd prefer, but even undies can change your body shape and, if you're going to start being comfortable in your own skin, maybe it's time to take the plunge and go for the Full Monty.

'IF YOU CAN BEAR IT, TAKE OFF ALL YOUR CLOTHES…IT'S TIME TO TAKE THE PLUNGE AND GO FOR THE FULL MONTY'

What Is Your Body Shape?

There are **four main body shapes** and a million other peculiarities in between. You might hate your knobbly knees or your droopy shoulders, love your slender ankles or swan-like neck, and it will be useful to remember these points. But, as the song says, '*You've got to accentuate the positive, eliminate the negative, latch on to the affirmative, don't mess with Mr In-Between!*'

Pear

This is the most common shape for women. Your upper body will be smaller than your hips and your widest parts will be your thighs and bottom. Learn how to make the most of your more delicate shoulders and shapely arms.

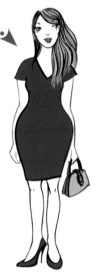

Hourglass

Take a bow, you Marilyn Monroe lookalike, you. Hourglass girls have nipped-in waists and voluptuous tops and bottoms. You should be sticking to fitted clothes to show off your curves.

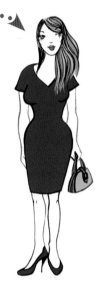

Apple

If you feel like you have thickened around your middle, giving you a rounded look, then you are an apple. With little waist definition, it can be tricky to find clothes to suit, but don't forget your boobs and legs!

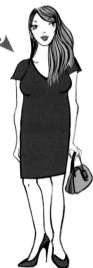

Athletic

You go straight up and down without bothering with the curvy bits. Athletic types can carry off most styles fabulously (think of models) but you may need a little help achieving a sexier, more feminine look.

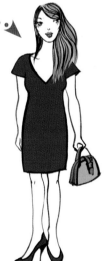

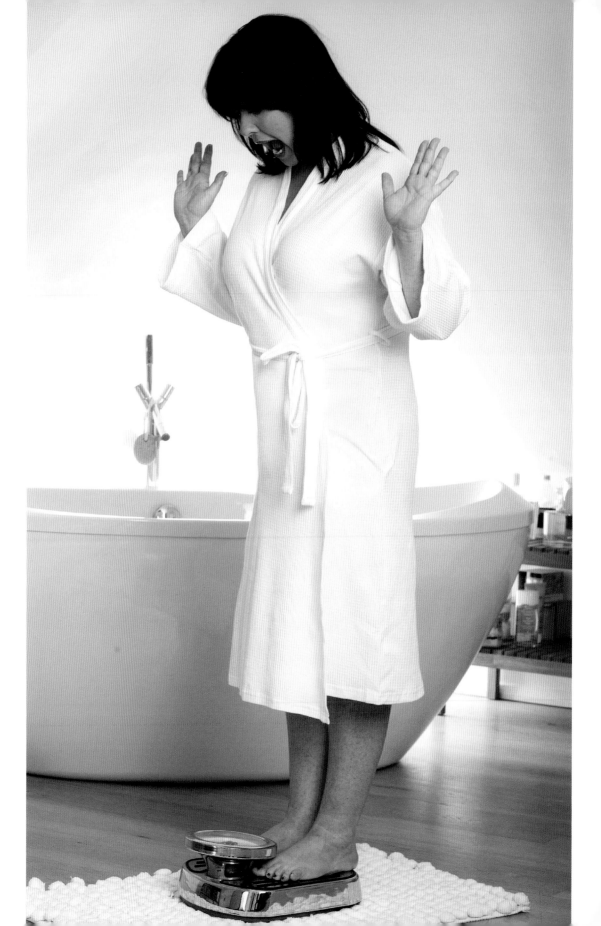

WEIGHT

EVERY WOMAN I KNOW IS HER WORST CRITIC, SO SHE DOESN'T NEED A CHART TO TELL HER IF SHE'S A FEW POUNDS OVERWEIGHT. IF YOUR JEANS FEEL TIGHT, YOUR BUTTONS ARE BURSTING AND YOU'VE NO ENERGY, YOU KNOW YOU'VE GOT TO GO EASY ON THE DOUGHNUTS. BUT SOMETIMES *FEELING* FAT HAS NOTHING TO DO WITH WHAT YOU ARE EATING. MAYBE IT'S DOWN TO YOUR MOOD, YOUR WORK SITUATION OR YOUR LACK OF CONFIDENCE?

As I have learned, eating sensibly, upping the exercise and learning to love yourself a little more will work wonders, but if you really want to know if you are overweight, here's how to do it. It's quite complicated and you'll find calculators on many internet websites if you want someone else to do the maths bit for you.

1. Work out your height in metres and multiply the figure by itself.

2. Measure your weight in kilograms.

3. Divide the answer to step 2 by the answer you got to step 1. For example, you might be 1.6m (5ft 3in) tall and weigh 65kg (10st 3lb). The calculation would then therefore be: 1.6 x 1.6 = 2.56. So your BMI would be: 65 ÷ 2.56 = 25.39.

UNDERWEIGHT:	less than 18.5
NORMAL WEIGHT:	18.5 to 24.9
OVERWEIGHT:	25 to 29.9
OBESE:	30 or greater

Don't panic if you fall into one of the last two categories. We'll look at ways of tackling this later on in the book.

HAIR

WHEN MY HAIR LOOKS GOOD, I FEEL FABULOUS. SHINY, SEXY HAIR THAT HAS BEEN CUT AND STYLED WELL CAN PICK A WOMAN UP LIKE NOTHING ELSE. TAKE A CLOSE LOOK AT YOUR HAIR AND ESTABLISH JUST WHAT TYPE YOU HAVE. LATER I'LL PASS ON SOME TIPS THAT WILL HELP YOU TREAT YOUR LOCKS WELL AND KEEP THEM LOOKING LOVELY.

What Is Your Hair Type?

Wait until the day after you've washed your hair and try the blot test:

- Dab a tissue onto your scalp and see how much oil is absorbed.
- If there is a dab of oil on the tissue, it means you have normal hair.
- If the tissue is clean, you have dry hair – this may be due to inactive oil glands or to nasties such as too much sun, harsh shampoos or chemicals.
- If the tissue is very oily, then your hair is greasy (but you didn't need me to tell you that, did you?). We'll look at ways to improve the condition of your hair later on in the book.

So now you know if your hair is dry, normal or greasy, you need to identify the other problems that could be ruining your crowning glory.

'SHINY, SEXY HAIR THAT HAS BEEN CUT AND STYLED WELL CAN PICK A WOMAN UP LIKE NOTHING ELSE'

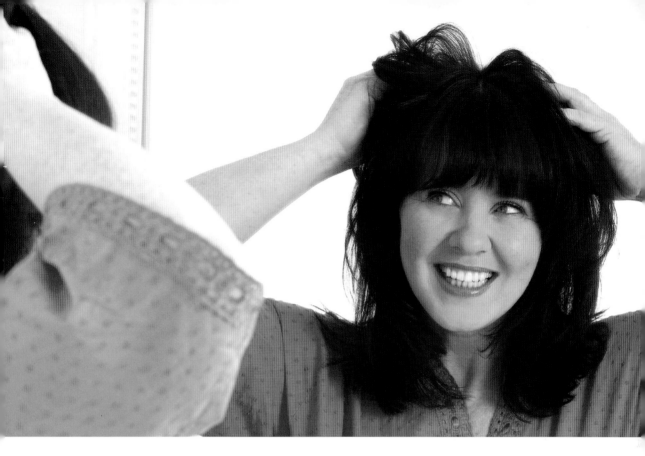

● *Thinning Hair*

Sweep your hair into a ponytail and see how many times you can loop a small covered hairband round it. Healthy hair should be thick enough to stay in place in just a couple of loops.

● *Damaged Hair*

It's a tough world out there, and extreme weather conditions, straightening irons, hairdryers and bleach will all leave their mark on your poor locks. If your hair never looks shiny, has very little volume or has split ends, then it's suffering and needs some TLC.

● *Dull and Lifeless Hair*

Hair health starts inside the body with what you eat and drink. If your hair is dull, it's time to look at your diet.

● *Dandruff*

This is another problem that can be helped along by eating the right foods. More about this later on.

EXERCISE

I'VE LOST WEIGHT ON NUMEROUS OCCASIONS BEFORE. I'VE TRIED EVERY FAD DIET GOING AND I'VE TRIED TO CHANGE THE WAY I LOOK JUST BY CONTROLLING WHAT GOES INTO MY MOUTH.

But you know what? Much as I hate to say it, the only way to keep the weight off is to combine sensible eating with increased exercise. You don't have to join an expensive gym or pound the streets. Anything that gets the heart racing and strengthens your muscles is fine.

So, when was the last time you touched your toes or got out of breath? Do you even own a pair of trainers? Take these quick tests to see how fit (or otherwise) you are. And don't worry, if you can clean the house without panting or dance all night without the use of an oxygen tank, you're already on your way. Don't forget to have a chat with your GP first, though, before starting any new exercise regime.

Test Your Upper-Body Strength

See how many push-ups you can do without collapsing – you can do it on bent knees if you'd prefer – then check the chart opposite to see if you fall into the acceptable range. Don't worry if you can't manage to reach this level; we'll look at how to improve your fitness levels later on.

AGE	PUSH-UPS	
• 20–9	• 17–33	✓
• 30–9	• 12–24	✓
• 40–9	• 8–19	✓
• 50–9	• 6–14	✓
• 60+	• 3–4	✓

Aerobic Fitness

AGE	DISTANCE (IN MILES)	
• 20 – 9	• 1.33	✔
• 30 – 9	• 1.27	✔
• 40 – 9	• 1.21	✔
• 50 – 9	• 1.13	✔
• 60+	• 1.07	✔

Discovering how far you can walk at a fast pace, jog or run in twelve minutes is a good way of testing your aerobic fitness. Warm up first, then using a pedometer that gives you distance as well as steps, or by using a length of pavement that can be measured later in your car, travel as far as you can in a strictly timed twelve minutes. Don't push yourself, just do what feels comfortable, then check the chart opposite to see if you fall into your age range. Keep a record of your results and test yourself again once you've started a fitness routine to see if you've improved.

STRESS

I WANT TO SPEND SOME TIME AT THE END OF THIS BOOK LOOKING AT HOW STRESS LEVELS CAN AFFECT OUR LIVES AND HOW, BY LEARNING TO RELAX, WE CAN BECOME MORE BEAUTIFUL, OUTSIDE AND IN.

Would you say you are living a stressful life? If you're a busy mum or a working woman, then it's quite likely that you are. I know I have to take precious time out every now and again to calm things down and give myself a break.

Think carefully about the last three days. Was there a time during those three days when you totally lost it? Or a moment when you felt completely overwhelmed by the jobs you had to do? Did you hear yourself saying 'yes' when your brain was screaming 'No!' Sound familiar? Then make sure you read Chapter 8 and learn how to feel good inside as well as looking fabulous outside. So now you know yourself a little better, let's begin…

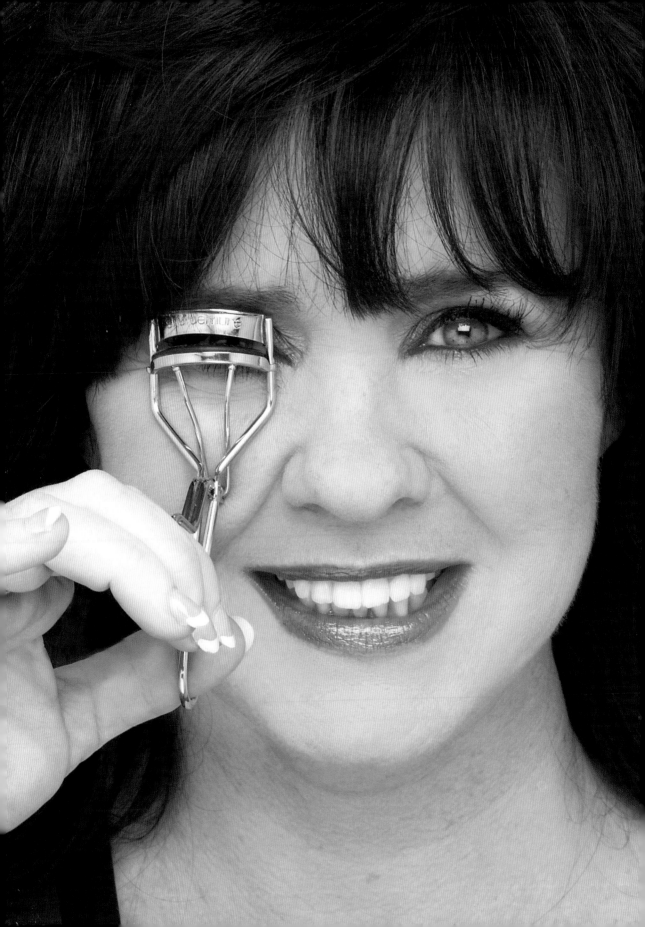

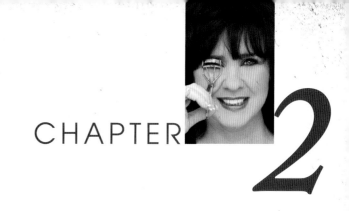
*Don't it make my
brown eyes blue....*

YOUR FACE
AND MAKE-UP

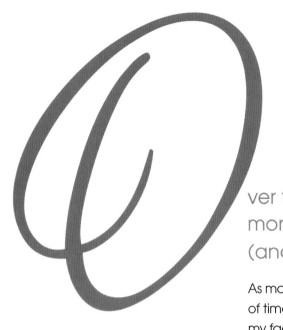ver the years I've had to sit in front of more mirrors than I've had hot dinners (and that's saying something).

As make-up artists have worked their magic, I've had plenty of time to study my own features: the oval-to-round shape of my face, my pale, freckly skin tone and combination complexion. I know my face like the back of my hand.

When I was a teenager I agonised over my appearance just like everyone else. I never had acne, but every now and then huge, disgusting spots with massive heads would suddenly erupt. My sisters used to hold me down to try to squeeze them. I often had to go on stage and face the audience knowing that only a layer of make-up stood between them and a meat-feast pizza. Thank God for foundation!

Thankfully my skin improved with age. I still get the occasional eruption, but providing I remember to cleanse and moisturise, I'm generally rewarded with a spot-free existence.

'YOUR FACE IS THE FIRST THING PEOPLE NOTICE ABOUT YOU'

My mum, Maureen, had beautiful skin. Despite not having a beauty regime she never had a wrinkle, not even in her eighties. It's hard to believe but I swear it's true. She was in showbiz too and I remember her telling us she had to take off the old greasepaint make-up with margarine! After she retired she only ever used soap and water, yet she never had a blemish. I think not drinking alcohol and not

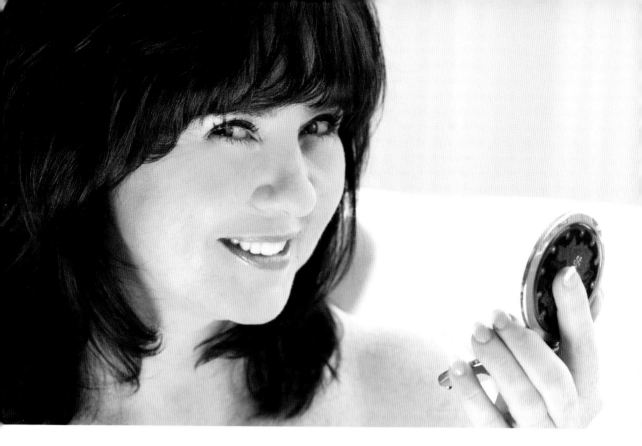

smoking helped enormously, that and being addicted to fruit. She'd eat five oranges a day if she could get her hands on them.

Mercifully I seem to have inherited her genes. That said, I'm determined not to leave it to chance – I've seen the future, and I don't like it.

It was during filming for a television beauty special I made for ITV called *The Truth About...Eternal Youth* that an age-progression artist showed me how I could look in ten and twenty years' time. I went to London's Harley Street where the artist Auriole Prince enhanced wrinkles around my eyes...it was truly terrifying.

Don't get me wrong, I know we all have to get older and I'm not ready to resort to the surgeon's knife just yet, but seeing those images convinced me to take care of my face so that I can look younger for longer.

Your face is the first thing people notice about you, so it's important to aim for glowing skin, a clear complexion and clever use of make-up. And in this chapter that's exactly what we're going to learn how to do.

SKIN

AS I SAID EARLIER, I HAVE MY MUM TO THANK FOR MY RELATIVELY TROUBLE-FREE SKIN, SO OBVIOUSLY THE GENETIC CARDS WE'VE BEEN DEALT HAVE AN IMPORTANT INFLUENCE ON THE WAY WE LOOK.

But skin can be enhanced or damaged by many things – extreme weather or pollution, the food and drink we consume, the chemicals we put into our bodies and the stress we endure in our lives. We can control most of these factors – a matter we'll come to a little later on – but the very best thing we can do in the quest for facial loveliness is to cleanse and moisturise our skin first thing in the morning and last thing at night. Not just when we remember, or when we're not too tipsy or tired after a busy evening out. EVERY. SINGLE. TIME!

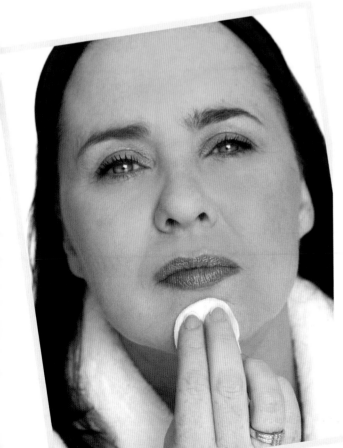

Cleansing

Think about what your poor face has to put up with during a typical day: grime from the environment, grease from make-up and the body's own gunk that is eliminated through the skin. It's obvious that a good cleansing routine will make you feel fresher and help the skin to breathe and recover.

WHICH ROUTINE SHOULD YOU CHOOSE?

The right cleanser for you is the one that leaves your face feeling clean and comfortable, and depending on your skin type, some will do a better job than others.

Removing the War Paint!

Before you cleanse your face you'll need to take away the day's lipstick and eye make-up. The skin around your eyes is the most delicate on your face and the first area where you'll notice wrinkles, so be gentle. Use your fingertips to apply make-up removal cream softly and then wipe away lightly with cotton wool. The same cream can be used on a tissue to wipe away lipstick too.

Normal Skin

Choose a cleansing milk or lotion that can be used with cotton wool or a gentle facial soap bar that rinses off with water.

Oily Skin

Again, you can use a rinse-off cleanser (oil-free if you can find it). If you're prone to the occasional outbreak of spots, a medicated face wash may help.

Dry Skin

Use a creamy, moisturising cleanser or a milk or lotion that isn't perfumed, and avoid drying extracts such as peppermint.

Sensitive Skin

Always use a hypo-allergenic cleanser so as not to aggravate or dry out the skin.

Toning

Lots of beauty books will tell you that toning is a vital stage between cleansing and moisturising, and it's true that a toner will take away any last bits of cleanser and tighten up your pores. But life's too short to follow *three* must-do routines, and if there's one bit I skip, toning is it. Toners can be harsh, so that's another reason I don't bother, plus it's just more expense. However, if you like the feel of squeaky-clean skin, try one of my home-made recipes at the end of this chapter as they will cost you almost nothing.

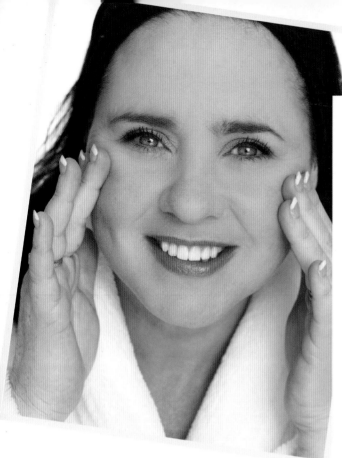

Moisturising

If I could only take one beauty product with me to a desert island it would have to be moisturiser. Every day our skin is dried by the elements and the effects of even the gentlest of cleansers, and it's important to replace as much moisture as possible if we are to beat off the early signs of ageing and stop wrinkles in their tracks.

Daytime moisturiser should be lighter and include an SPF (sun protection factor) of at least 15, whereas night-time moisturisers can be thicker, or richer, as they're absorbed while you snooze.

Normal Skin

Most moisturisers will suit you, but go for the lightest version that leaves your skin feeling comfortable and remember not to put too much on as this can clog your pores.

Oily Skin

Even oily skin needs to be moisturised, but steer clear of greasy lotions. Choose a water-based, oil-free brand to help replenish moisture.

Dry Skin

Choose a creamy, oil-based moisturiser. Generally speaking, the drier your skin, the thicker the moisturiser you should use.

Sensitive Skin

Go for a fragrance-free, hypo-allergenic moisturiser. You could first dab a little on the sensitive area behind your ear to make sure it doesn't irritate your skin.

Exfoliating

I started using rubs and scrubs to get rid of dead skin cells on my body years before I realised exfoliation was a great treat for my face, too. Most exfoliating creams use either natural rough particles or smoother, man-made granules, which are excellent for sensitive types. They even out the tone of your skin and leave your face feeling smoother, lighter and brighter. But don't overdo it. Normal skin needs exfoliating no more than once a week and dry skin will dry out even further if you do this more than once a fortnight.

Don't get carried away with expensive facial scrubs either. A gentle rub with a clean, dry face flannel can leave your skin feeling really good, or take a look at some of my home-made scrubs at the end of the chapter.

Steaming

My teenage mates and I used to spend hours with our heads under towels and our faces over steaming bowls of water, emerging like lobsters ready for a really good blackhead-squeezing session!

Steaming is a natural and cheap way of giving your face a really good cleanse. The heat will make you sweat out impurities and improve circulation to leave your face feeling as soft as a baby's bottom. You'll find expensive gadgets in the shops, but all you really need is a bowl of freshly boiled water and a clean towel to cover your head.

Keep your face about 30cm above the water and stay there for no more than ten minutes. Afterwards, rinse your face with warm water, dab with a clean towel and moisturise.

If you have sensitive skin, you might find the heat irritates it, so try a shorter test run first. If you have normal or oily skin, then a steaming treatment two or three times a week should be fine; limit it to once a week if your skin is dry.

ROLLING BACK THE YEARS

EVEN IF I CAN OCCASIONALLY KID MYSELF THAT I'M NOT *REALLY* IN MY FORTIES, AS A WOMAN ON THE TELLY I'M NEVER ALLOWED TO FORGET HOW OLD I ACTUALLY AM. WHEN I WAS COMPETING ON *DANCING ON ICE*, THE VIEWERS WERE REPEATEDLY REMINDED HOW 'PLUCKY COLEEN' WAS ALMOST TWICE THE AGE OF SOME OF THE OTHER FEMALE CONTESTANTS. CHARMING!

There is enormous emphasis put on the way women look and we get judged by our age and appearance constantly. It's not surprising then that there's a multi-million-pound industry out there dedicated to helping us roll back the years.

Up until our late twenties most of us will have laughed at skincare routines and ignored the hundreds of lotions and potions on the shop shelves. What we should have been concentrating on was keeping our skin clean and slapping on the sunscreen. If you're lucky enough to be in your twenties now, then think to the future…and if not, tell your daughters.

Once we hit our thirties the damage done by the sun and other lifestyle nasties starts to show in the form of fine lines and wrinkles. It's a sad fact that the older we get, the more pots of beauty cream we will own, and it's about now that you might start thinking about eye creams and anti-ageing treatments.

In our forties the laughter lines will have become deeper creases and our skin will be starting to lose its ability to spring back into place. Our pores will look bigger and those face packs and expensive creams will begin to look even more attractive.

By the time we enter our fifties and sixties the life we have lived is written all over our face. Slap! On goes the night-time gunk and thoughts may even turn to a bit of Botox or a trip to the plastic surgeon. What a pity we didn't take a little more care of our skin all those years ago…

I know we can't really turn back the clock, but it's never too late to protect your face from the sun. It's the greatest enemy we have in the battle for beauty and I make no apologies for repeating: use a moisturiser or foundation with an SPF of no less than 15.

Meanwhile there are hundreds of anti-ageing creams to try. When I made *The Truth About…Eternal Youth,* I road-tested the most ridiculously priced potions, and I can't say they did anything different to my usual moisturiser. So don't be fooled by a hefty price tag or designer label.

If you are going to spend your hard-earned cash on skincare products, however, there are some ingredients worth looking out for. Retinol, a form of vitamin A, is said to be a brilliant anti-ageing product because it encourages the growth of collagen and boosts cell renewal. Another scientific name to look for is peptides, which are little particles of protein that help repair damaged skin cells.

Also, look out for skincare products containing antioxidants, which repair damage caused by free radicals. Sorry to get technical here, but trust me, too many free radicals are bad news for your skin. To get the benefits of antioxidants in your skincare products, look for the ingredients vitamins A, C and E and coenzyme Q10.

It's also worth looking out for products containing the essential fatty acids Omega 3 and 6. The experts say they do wonders for your skin, nails and hair.

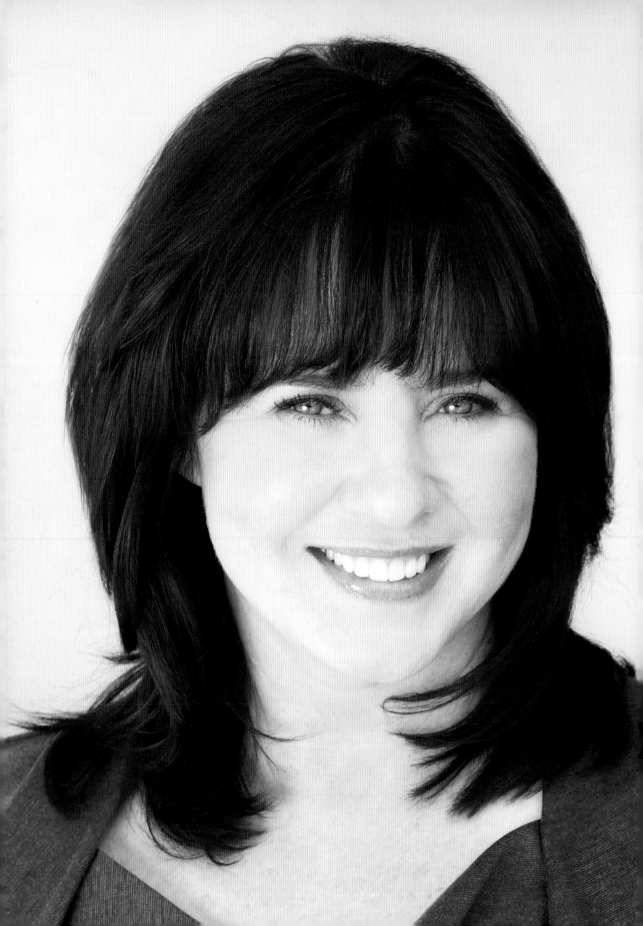

My Bad Habit

There are a hundred good reasons why I shouldn't smoke – my kids, my husband, my health, my finances – but the one that stares me in the face each day is the effect it has on my skin.

It's not rocket science – I know my complexion would be a million times better if I didn't smoke – but unfortunately it's a habit I've had for years and so far it's proven impossible to give up. I will do it, I know I will. Every day I come closer to it and it's only a matter of time. So watch this space and some day soon I'll be fag-free!

A Cut Above?

Years ago, if you wanted to look better you'd assess your diet and lifestyle and you'd work hard to make changes. Nowadays, though, people want immediate results and consequently some go down the surgical route. And it's not just for tighter tums and bigger boobs – facelifts and Botox are becoming almost the norm. I find this obsession with anti-ageing surgery terrifying – have you noticed how women who have fiddled with their faces are all starting to look the same?

When I made The Truth About…Eternal Youth *I was offered a nip and tuck and I have to admit I did think about it, but only for about ten seconds. For a start I'm a coward, and as mum to Ciara, Jake and Shane Junior I just couldn't risk being put to sleep for an operation that wasn't essential. But also, much as I want to look youthful, I'm quite proud of my laughter lines. They are a sign that I have truly lived, and laughed, for a great part of my life.*

I would never judge anyone for having surgery or Botox, but I wish women would start feeling better about the way they look rather than constantly trying to make themselves look like someone else.

FEED YOUR FACE

NO, NOT WITH CHOCOLATE BISCUITS BUT WITH FOOD AND DRINK THAT CAN, QUITE LITERALLY, FEED THE SKIN ON YOUR FACE.

Even the world's most expensive skin lotion is powerless to fight the damage caused by a bad diet. And, luckily for us, a good diet can be so beneficial it can save us spending a fortune on some fancy promise-in-a-pot.

The best diet for sensational skin is one that includes all the nutrients needed for good health – protein, carbs, fats, vitamins and minerals. Eat loads of fresh fruit and vegetables, yoghurt, honey, vegetable oils, seeds, nuts and grains. Good sources of protein include oily fish, white meat and, for vegetarians, soya beans and tofu. Remember also to drink lots of water – eight glasses a day if you can manage it – to purify the system and keep your skin clear and your eyes sparkling.

You can get an added hit of vitamin C by starting your morning off with a mug of hot water and the juice of half a lemon. It's a trick I learned years ago and it really sets me up for the day ahead. Plus your skin will get a double boost from the hydrating effect of the water and the detoxing effect of the lemon.

Meanwhile, don't forget the baddies in your diet. Alcohol and coffee will absorb moisture from your face and too much sugar will damage protein molecules in your skin, reducing its elasticity and leading to premature ageing. That's not to say you can never again enjoy a glass of wine or a bar of chocolate; just do it in moderation.

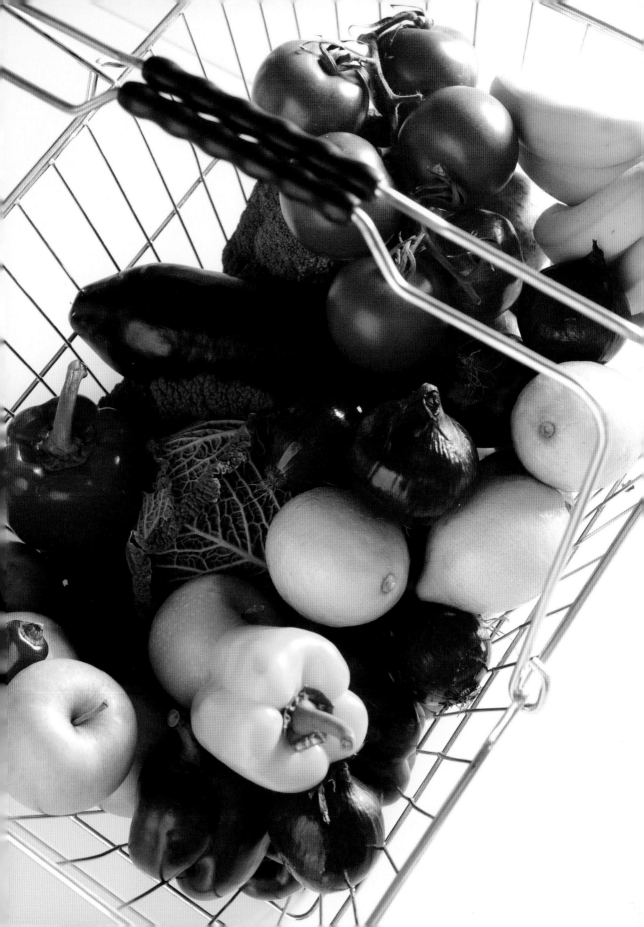

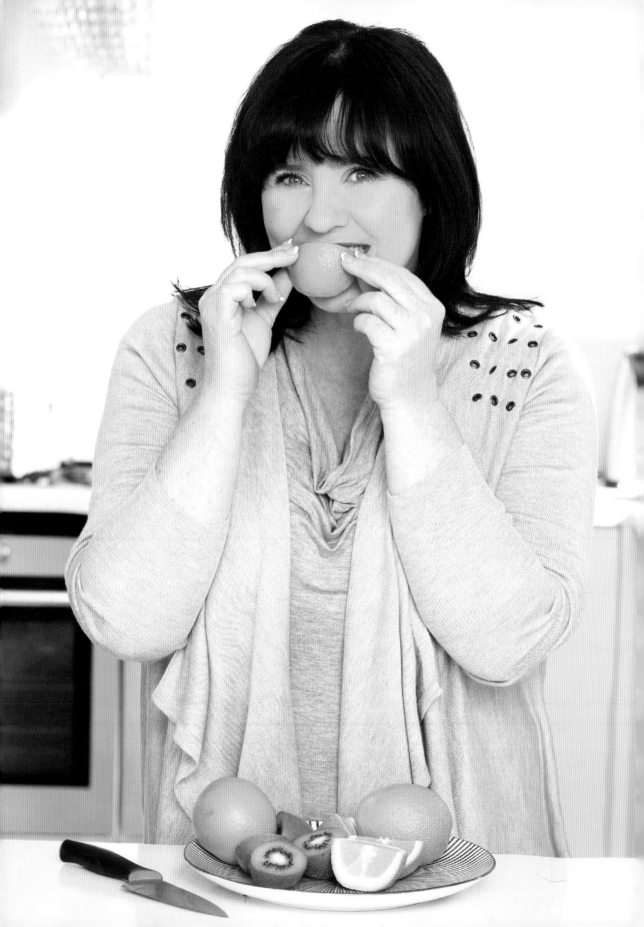

My Top Skin-Friendly Foods

Remember how I told you about the various vitamins to look out for in skincare products? Well, you can also find these skincare heroes in the foods you eat.

1 Anything containing the antioxidant **VITAMIN A** will encourage new skin to grow and keep your complexion looking young. I get mine from liver, eggs and milk.

2 **VITAMIN B2** helps skin develop and is said to really make it glow, and it can be found in yoghurt, spinach, peas…and Marmite!

3 I get my hit of **VITAMIN C**, which encourages the production of collagen for smooth skin as well as being an antioxidant, from oranges, grapefruit, blackcurrants, blueberries, broccoli, kiwi and sweet potato.

4 **VITAMIN E** is the vitamin most often seen on the labels of skincare products and is said to reduce wrinkles. I get mine from avocados, tomatoes, olive oil and wholemeal bread.

5 For **OMEGA 3**, which is good for the joints as well as promoting supple skin, I love oily fish such as salmon, sardines and fresh tuna.

6 **ZINC**-rich foods such as liver, sardines, prawns, sweet potatoes, bananas and Brazil nuts will repair skin damage, leaving skin soft and supple.

7 Finally, **IRON** will improve your skin tone, and with pale skin like mine that's important. I make sure I regularly eat lean red meat, eggs and leafy green vegetables – I love spinach, which is a great source of iron – and I always have dried apricots, almonds and Brazil nuts close by to snack on. Cocoa also contains iron, so that's one reason not to feel guilty when you tuck into a chocolate bar. Just make sure it's dark chocolate with at least 70 per cent cocoa and don't forget to stop after one or two squares.

BRIGHT EYES

I'M A SUCKER FOR A MAN WITH NICE EYES. BLUE, BROWN, HAZEL, I DON'T REALLY CARE, JUST FLASH ME A PAIR OF TWINKLY EYES AND I'M PUTTY!

Us ladies are lucky in that we can enhance what we've been given by using clever make-up tricks. But you won't always have time to reach for the mascara and that's why it's important to know the basics.

For instance, did you know that rabbits really do know a thing or two about eating the right foods for good eyesight? Yes, carrots are great for healthy eyes, as are most fresh fruit and green vegetables.

Looking like a panda? If you don't get enough sleep then dark circles will form under your eyes. What's actually happening is that lack of sleep is making the rest of your face paler and enhancing the dark area under your eyes, but whatever the reason, it's not a great look, so make sure you get your full eight hours.

Dull or bloodshot eyes can be caused by dehydration, so don't forget to drink plenty of water. And don't wait until you're thirsty – by then you're already dehydrated.

Too much time in front of a computer screen is also bad for you and will make your eyes look and feel extremely tired. If your job involves sitting in front of a screen, make sure you take a break every fifteen or twenty minutes.

And finally a word about eyebrows. A well-shaped brow can do as much for your face as an eyelift, so learn how to keep yours nicely trimmed and shaped.

TRY THIS PENCIL TEST TO SEE IF YOURS ARE TOO THICK:

- Hold a pencil along one side of your nose – you shouldn't see any stray brows past the inside edge of the pencil.

- Then, keeping the pencil next to your nose, tilt it to the outside corner of your eye:
– that's where your eyebrow should stop.

- Use a decent pair of tweezers to pluck away any stray hairs on either side of this, then clean up the area beneath your brow. Don't go mad, though. You don't want arched eyebrows like Mr Spock, just tidy-looking brows that frame your eyes beautifully.

If you find plucking painful, try doing it after a bath or shower when the skin is warmer and your pores are open to let the hair out more easily. If you're really hopeless when it comes to looking after your brows, you could book yourself in for a professional pluck from an expert on a make-up counter. Or ask about threading, waxing or laser hair-removal treatments at your local beauty salon.

LOVELY LIPS

IT'S THE SKIN YOU USE TO KISS YOUR CHILDREN, AND YOUR PARTNER, SO KEEP YOUR LIPS AS SOFT AS SILK AND IN GREAT CONDITION.

The lips have no sebaceous glands – in other words they don't produce any natural oils – so it's important to keep them artificially moisturised, especially in extreme weather conditions.

You don't need expensive lip creams – a cheapo ChapStick or some Vaseline will do the trick just as well, especially when slathered on at night before you go to sleep.

If your lips are especially dry, you could try applying a little lip balm or cream first, then brushing them gently with a soft toothbrush. This will remove any flaky patches and help the moisturiser be absorbed into your skin.

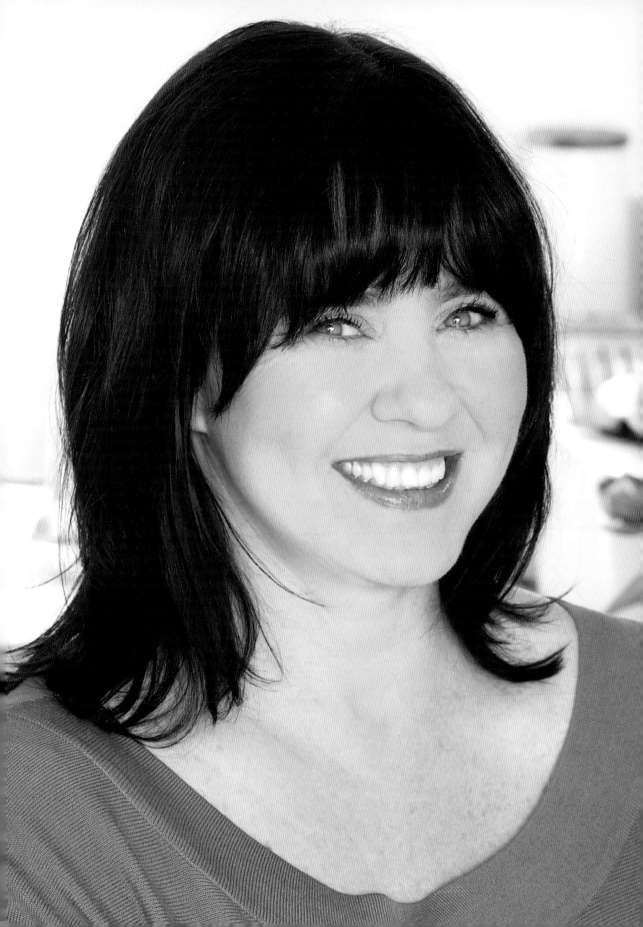

TIP-TOP TEETH

WHEN I MEET AMERICAN CELEBRITIES ON *LOOSE WOMEN* I'M ALWAYS ASTONISHED BY THEIR SPARKLING WHITE TEETH (HONESTLY, SOMETIMES YOU NEED TO WEAR SUNGLASSES).

Our cousins across the Pond are obsessed with straight, blindingly white teeth and think we're mad settling for our more natural look. I don't believe it's necessary to lose sleep over having a perfect set, but I do think it's important to look after what you've got and to keep your teeth clean and healthy. Not only will they look more attractive, it will save you a lot of pain and expense later on.

To this end, brush at least twice a day, floss daily and make sure you have regular check-ups with your dentist, where you can ask for tips on cleaning and brushes. Tea, coffee, red wine and smoking all stain tooth enamel, so think about avoiding these things if you're particularly worried. Or try brushing with one of the many whitening toothpastes on the market. They won't change the colour of your tooth enamel, but they can get rid of unsightly stains.

For truly sparkling white teeth you could go for a professional dental whitening treatment, but this will set you back a lot of money. You can buy DIY treatments in the shops, but make sure you read and follow the instructions extremely carefully. Some kits contain mild acids while others don't contain enough whitening products to make a difference. If in doubt, always look for the **British Dental Health Foundation-**approved logo.

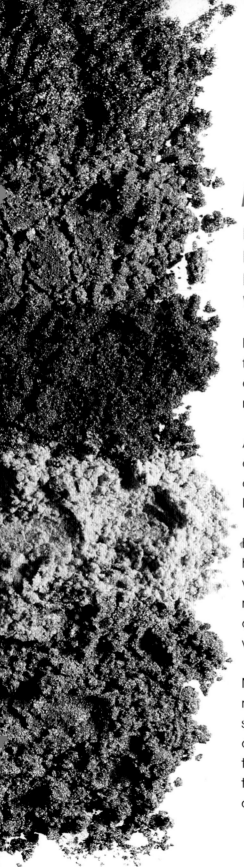

MAKE-UP

I WEAR MAKE-UP EVERY DAY – EVEN WHEN I'M IN THE HOUSE I'LL USE CONCEALER, MASCARA, BLUSHER AND LIPSTICK SO I DON'T SCARE MYSELF WHEN I LOOK IN THE MIRROR!

But I don't spend a fortune on it. I use my mascara until it's fit for the dustbin and I'll scrape the last bit of lipstick out of a favourite tube. In short, I only buy new stuff when there's nothing left in my make-up bag.

At most, I'll spend five minutes putting make-up on. I'm always in a mad rush and I don't have time to mess around. Besides, after thirty-plus years of slapping it on I know where it goes and what to do with it.

Even if I've got a big night out ahead I can shower, do my hair and put on my make-up in forty minutes. And they say women take a long time to get ready! I've seen enough miracles worked by make-up artists to know that a little concealer or lippy can transform anyone. I really do think we're luckier than men in that respect.

My earliest experiences of make-up involved watching my sisters get themselves ready to go on stage. I loved seeing all the pots and paints and watching how they could turn themselves into glamorous performers with the stroke of a brush. It wasn't long before I was nicking their stuff and practising on my own features, and now my daughter Ciara is doing the same thing.

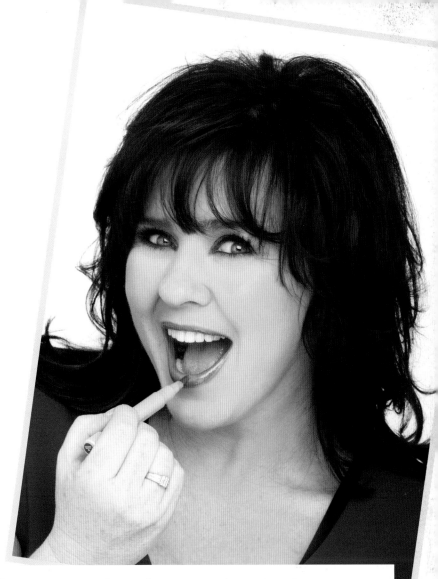

'WHY NOT ASK FOR A MAKE-UP LESSON AS A GIFT THIS CHRISTMAS? THEY CAN TEACH YOU PROFESSIONAL TRICKS AND ADVISE ON THE BEST COLOURS FOR YOU'

You've probably been applying your own make-up for years and wonder why you need to learn new tricks at this stage in your life. Well, just as wearing the same hairstyle for years can date you, so using the same colour eyeshadow or shade of blusher can seem old-fashioned. You need to move with the times.

I'm going to pass on a few tips I've learned over the years, but what you really need to do is grab a few precious moments to experiment. Why not ask for a make-up lesson as a gift this Christmas? You'll find make-up artists advertising in the phone book and local newspaper, and they can teach you professional tricks and advise on the best colours and products for you. Don't forget the cosmetic counters of department stores either. If you can stand being the centre of attention in the middle of a busy shop, you'll find beauty experts ready and willing to give you a new look.

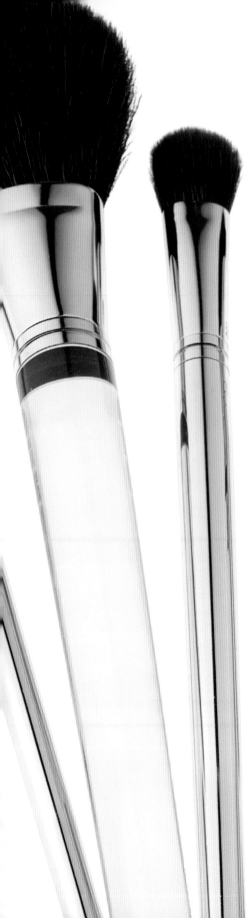

Tools of the Trade

A bad workman always blames his tools, so make sure you're using the right ones. Don't go mad and spend a lot of money; buy wisely and your equipment should last a long time. Use a gentle shampoo to ensure your brushes aren't a breeding ground for bacteria and keep your tools in a clean make-up bag or box. I admit I'm a bit of a make-up-bag slut and can forget to clean it out for ages. Only us women know how revolting a neglected make-up bag can be.

Depending on how you apply your make-up – and some prefer to use their fingers instead of sponges and brushes – you'll need the following:

⟶ *A soft sponge (natural or man-made)*

⟶ *Tweezers*

⟶ *Eyelash curlers*
   (they look like torture but can make a huge difference)

⟶ *Eyeshadow brushes*
   (keep a few for different colours and widths)

⟶ *Eyeliner brush*

⟶ *Pencil sharpener for eyeliners and lipliners*

⟶ *Large blusher brush (I like a really huge one!)*

⟶ *Lip brush*

⟶ *Cotton wool or a compact puff for powder*

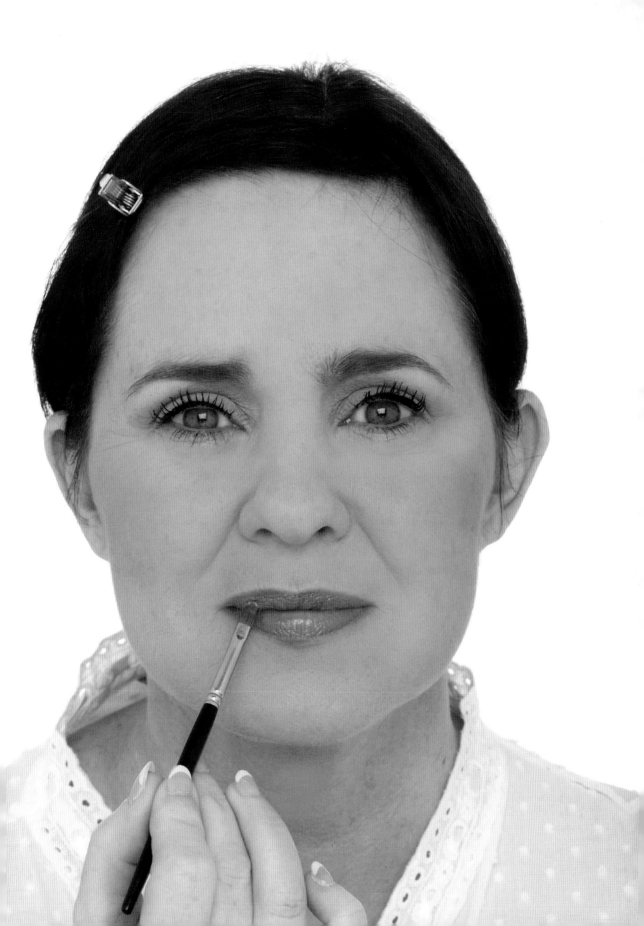

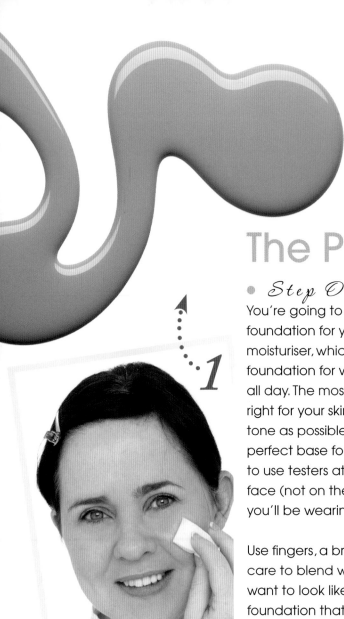

'IT'S ESSENTIAL TO FIND A SHADE THAT'S RIGHT FOR YOUR SKIN'

The Perfect Base

• *Step One, Foundation*

You're going to have to experiment to find the perfect foundation for you. There's a huge range, from tinted moisturiser, which is often all I use, to heavier cake foundation for when you need your 'face' to stay in place all day. The most essential thing is to find a shade that's right for your skin. It should be as close to your own skin tone as possible to leave you with a natural-looking, perfect base for the rest of your make-up. Don't be afraid to use testers at the beauty counter. Dab a little on your face (not on the back of your hand: that's not where you'll be wearing it!) and check it outside in natural light.

Use fingers, a brush or a damp sponge to apply and take care to blend well into your neck and hairline – you don't want to look like you're wearing a mask. Freshen up foundation that's been on for a few hours with a fingertip of moisturiser, especially under the eyes. And don't forget your SPF – if it's not in your skincare products, use a foundation with an SPF of 15 or more.

When choosing your foundation, think about your skin type. If you have dry skin, choose one that's oil-based; if you have oily skin, you'll be better off with water-based make-up, or try a mineral powder foundation that you brush on. Remember, too, that there are foundations specially formulated for sensitive skin.

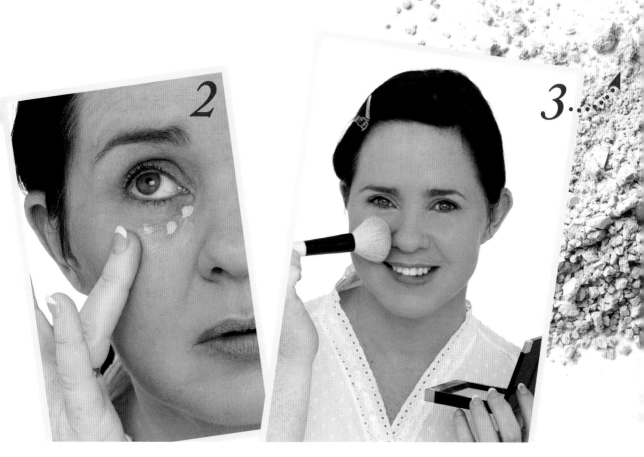

Step Two, Concealer

I wouldn't go anywhere without concealer as it covers up my blemishes, stops me looking like I have black eyes and makes me look less tired. Gently dab a creamy concealer on blemishes and under your eyes. Use your ring finger in this delicate area as it exerts the least pressure of all your fingers, and don't forget to put a spot on the inner corner of your eye to lighten the shadow of your nose. Concealers hiding blemishes should be thicker and closer to your skin colour, whereas those lifting shadows can be lighter both in consistency and colour. Personally, I just use the same stuff to save the time and expense of using two different products.

Step Three, Powder

If I'm in a real rush I don't always bother with powder, but I have to admit it does give your make-up the perfect finish. Certainly, make-up artists always use it to reduce shine and 'set' the foundation. You can choose from loose powder or solid powder in a compact (which always reminds me of my mum), but take care not to use too much as it can sit in fine lines and make you appear wrinkly – not a good look! Powder is great for a quick repair job in the middle of the day or on a night out.

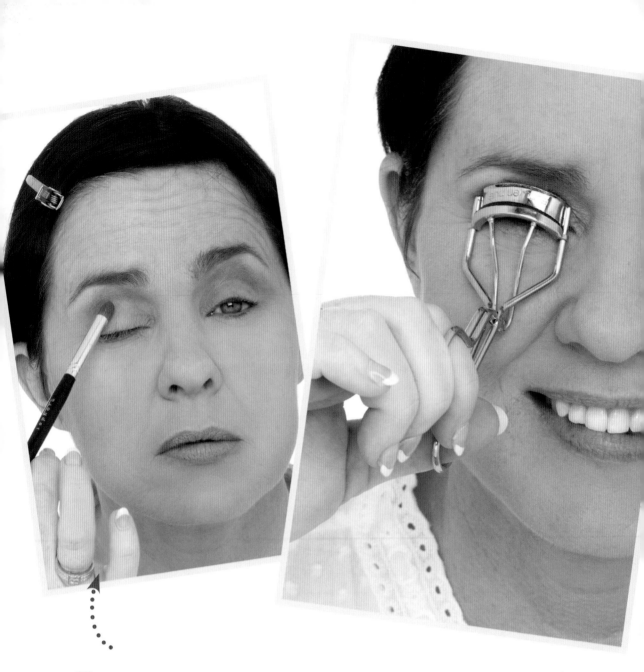

Eyes

This is the area I enjoy making up the most. Whether you opt for dark, dramatic eyes for a big night out or pretty, natural shades for daytime, eye make-up is perfect for making a statement. It's a good idea to do your eyes first then, using a baby wipe, clear away any dropped eyeshadow or smudged mascara from your cheeks before doing the rest of your make-up.

1 Using your fingers or an eyeshadow brush, sweep a base colour over your entire eye area. Choose a neutral shade close to your skin colour or just use your face powder.

2 Brush on your main colour, this time covering only the eyelid.

3 Apply a slightly darker colour along the crease of your eye socket and use your finger or a brush to blend it well.

4 Use a lighter eyeshadow on your brow bone to highlight the eye. Avoid pearly eyeshadow in this area – you don't want to look like you've time-travelled back to the Eighties.

5 Carefully line the eyes using an eyeliner pencil, liquid eyeliner or, if your eyes are smaller, a tiny brush with a little of the darker eyeshadow you've already used. Outlining the outer edges only will make your eyes look bigger. If you're aiming for a more natural look, line just the upper lid and apply under the bottom lashes for a dramatic effect. If you're getting ready for a party or a big night out, why not use a glittery liner – you're never too old to sparkle!

6 When I'm going on TV or on stage, I use a kohl pencil on the bottom inside rim of my eyes as it gives a really glam look.

7 Now for the eyelash curlers. You can buy eyelash curlers quite cheaply and use them to 'open up' the eyes before applying mascara. Gently clamp them onto your top lashes for a few seconds to curl and lengthen.

8 Finally, it's time to apply your mascara. Make sure you don't have too much on the wand, then sweep a light layer along the bottom lashes. Move on to the top lashes, brushing from root to tip. I only do this from underneath the lashes, but for a really dramatic effect you can apply it to the upper side, too. If you move the wand ever so slightly from side to side, your lashes will look even longer and you won't end up with clumpy mascara.

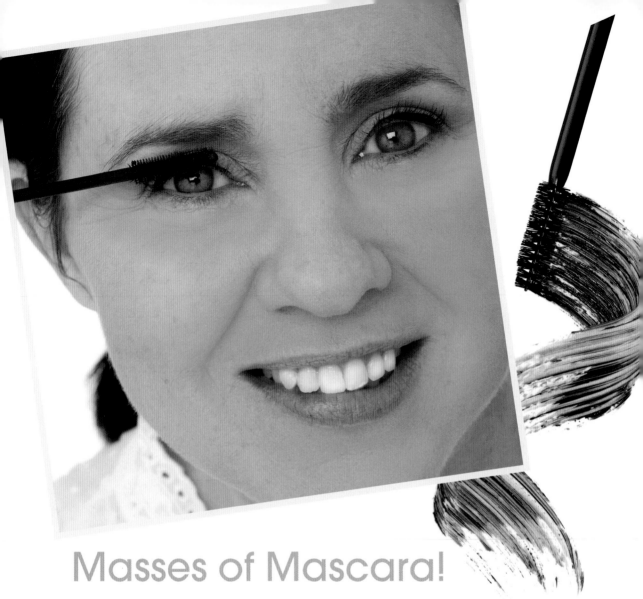

Masses of Mascara!

There are so many different types of mascara on the market that it's easy to give up and grab the one in the prettiest packaging. But don't despair, I have a couple of rules I always follow and I'm never seduced by expensive claims.

Rule 1: I never, ever use coloured mascara. For me, it's only ever black, which I think gives a classic, elegant look.

Rule 2: My eyelashes need thickening up a little, so I use a volumising mascara to give them more weight. A lengthening mascara will obviously make them longer and a waterproof mascara is good for weddings, hot sticky days and anytime you're likely to burst into tears.

'EVEN THE SUBTLEST OF FALSE EYELASHES WILL OPEN UP YOUR EYES AND GIVE YOU A FABULOUS AIR OF GLAMOUR'

Lashings of Lashes!

For a really special occasion I reach for the falsies. You can buy false eyelashes at any good cosmetics counter and you'll be amazed by their effect. You don't have to opt for the full Marilyn Monroe version; even the subtlest of falsies will open up your eyes and give you a fabulous air of glamour. You can buy full sets or individual lashes and often just a couple on the outside of the eye is enough.

Put them on your upper lid after your eyeshadow and before your eyeliner and mascara, carefully following the instructions on the packet. You'll be given a little tube of glue and it's probably a good idea to practise beforehand to avoid disasters.

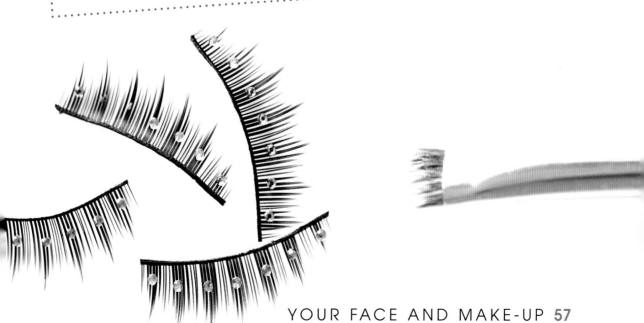

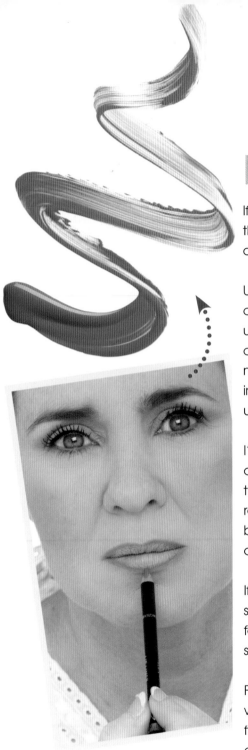

Lips

If you've gone for a dramatic look on the eyes, go easy on the lips and vice versa. Don't go crazy vamping up both areas or you'll end up looking like a street walker!

Use your foundation to give the lips a good base, then choose a lipliner to outline the shape of your mouth. Always use a liner that's the same colour as your lipstick – sometimes I cheat and use a small brush to line my lips with my lipstick. You never want to see the liner – that looks mad. Use a brush to fill in the lips, starting in the middle and working outwards, then use a tissue to blot any excess.

I've never followed any hard and fast rules when choosing a shade of lipstick – just experiment and wear what you think suits you (with the emphasis on *you* and your skin tone rather than your clothes – that just looks naff). You could use a brush to mix a couple of shades together to save buying a new lipstick.

If you're wearing foundation, I think you should always wear something on your lips, otherwise you'll look like you've forgotten something. But a slick of clear or pink lipgloss is sometimes all you need.

Finally, once you've put colour on your lips, that's where you want it to stay. To prevent it sticking to your teeth, put your finger in your mouth and slowly pull it out, taking with it any excess gloop. To stop it moving to your coffee mug or wineglass, discreetly run your tongue over the edge of the mug or glass: the saliva will form a barrier and keep your lipstick stuck to your lips.

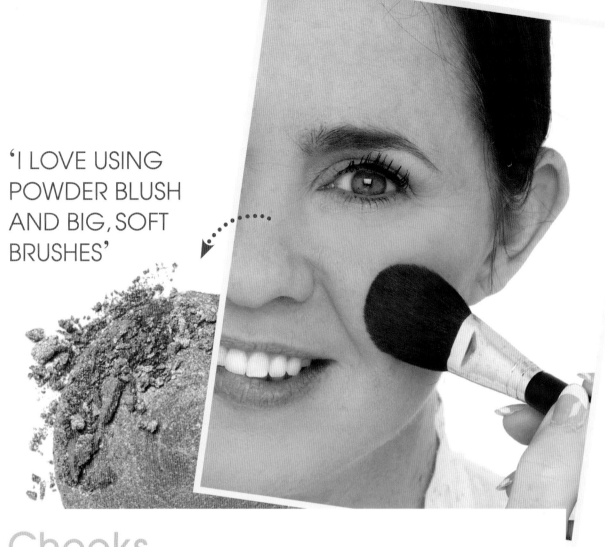

Cheeks

The last bit of make-up I apply is my blusher. A well-chosen, cleverly applied blusher can give you cheekbones, slim down your face and boost your colouring. If I don't wear blusher, people think I'm dying – my pale skin just cries out for it.

I love using powder blush and big, soft brushes, but you could use your fingertips to dot on and blend cream blush if you like. If you're using powder and a brush, gently blow the ends of the bristles before applying to make sure the colour isn't too heavy.

A good trick is to look in the mirror and smile. Find the fullest part of your cheeks (the apples) and sweep your brush over the area. If you don't have very defined cheekbones, you can add definition by using a blusher under the bone to make it stand out. But be careful, we're not aiming for the Adam Ant look here, so stripes are to be avoided!

Make-Up In Minutes

I'm very lucky that when I need to look my best I usually have someone on hand to sort me out. Professional make-up artists are magicians – did you see me on *Loose Women* without make-up that time? Not a pretty sight! But as a busy working mum I know it's just not practical to start each day with a full make-up routine.

HERE ARE A FEW TRICKS I'VE LEARNED TO HELP SAVE TIME AND MONEY:

- Find products that will do two jobs at once, such as powdered blusher you can use for your eyes and cheeks, or lip colour that doubles as a blusher.

- On the back of your hand mix together an SPF moisturiser and a foundation to give a sheer, creamy consistency. It will save time only having to apply one base.

- Plain old Vaseline is one of my favourite products. If I'm short on time, I use it to moisturise and gloss my lips, then dab a little on my cheeks for a dewy effect.

- If I don't have time for foundation and blusher, I use a bronzer on my brow, nose and chin for a healthy glow.

- I keep a little bottle of eye drops handy to wake me up if my eyes are feeling really tired.

- If I don't even have time to stand still in front of a mirror, I make sure I use clear lipgloss. I can do that with my eyes closed.

- Baby wipes are not just for baby: they are great for a quick once over when I don't have time to remove my make-up properly.

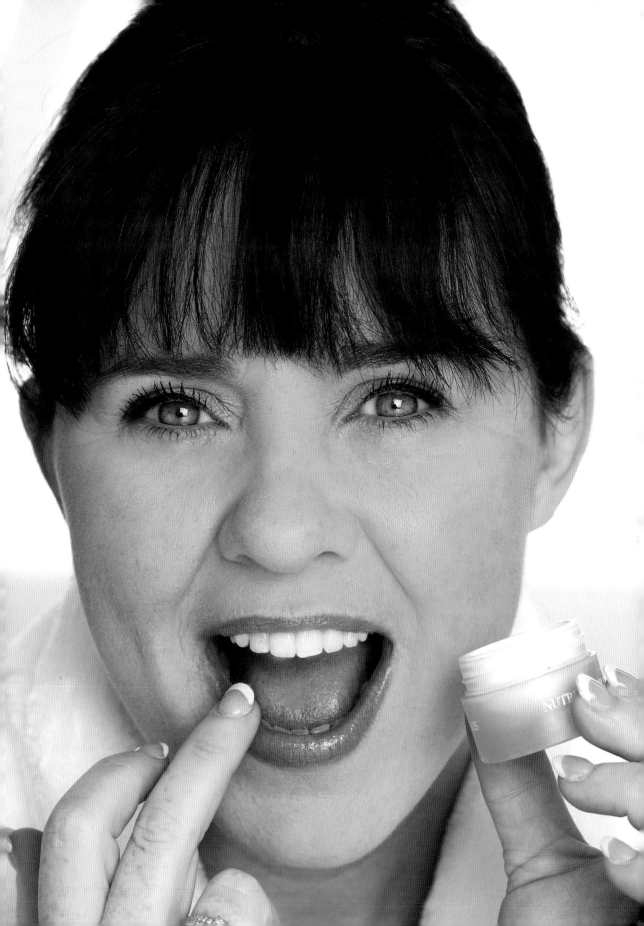

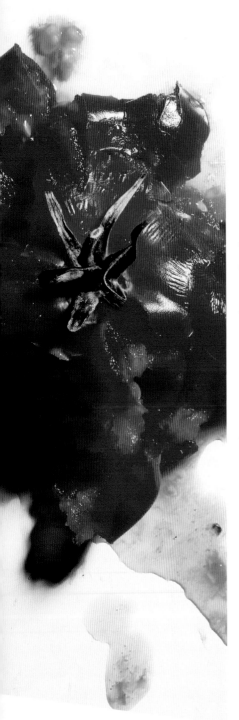

HELP YOURSELF FOR FREE

YOU DON'T HAVE TO SPEND LOTS OF MONEY ON YOUR SKINCARE AND DAILY BEAUTY ROUTINE; YOU'LL FIND ALL THE INGREDIENTS FOR THESE DIY TREATMENTS IN YOUR KITCHEN.

• *Cucumber Face Mask*
(TO PREVENT BLACKHEADS AND DRY SKIN)

Grate or blend a cucumber in a food processor. Apply over your face, eyes and neck and leave for up to twenty minutes. Rinse your face with warm water and pat dry.

• *Tomato Face Mask*
(TO REDUCE GREASINESS IN OILY SKIN)

Mash up a ripe, squashy tomato and apply to the skin on your face for fifteen to twenty minutes. Rinse with lukewarm water.

• *Apple and Honey Face Mask*
(FOR OILY SKIN OR SKIN PRONE TO SPOTS)

Finely grate one apple and mix with five tablespoons of runny honey. Smooth it over your face and leave for ten minutes. Rinse off with cool water.

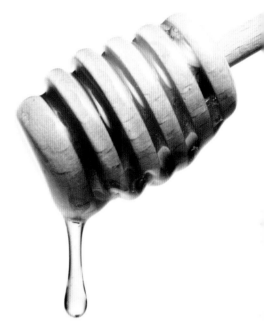

Avocado Face Mask
(TO CLEAN THE PORES AND MOISTURISE SKIN)

Peel and mash a ripe avocado, then smooth the pulp onto your face. Leave it for fifteen minutes, then rinse off with warm water.

Oatmeal Face Mask
(FOR OILY SKIN)

Mix a tablespoon of runny honey with one egg yolk, then stir in 60ml of oatmeal to make a soft paste. Apply the mask to the face and neck and leave for fifteen minutes. Rinse away with lukewarm water.

Honey Cleanser
(GOOD FOR CLEANSING AND LEAVING SKIN MOIST)

Mix one tablespoon of honey with two tablespoons of ground almonds and half a teaspoon of lemon juice. Rub onto the face and rinse off after five minutes with lukewarm water.

Sea-Salt Scrub
(TO REMOVE DRY SKIN AND TIGHTEN THE PORES)

Gently massage two tablespoons of coarse sea salt onto your wet face, taking care not to get it in your eyes. After two minutes rinse well and splash your face with cold water.

Sugar Scrub
(TO EXFOLIATE AND LEAVE SKIN FEELING SOFT)

Mix 400g of brown sugar with five tablespoons of milk and apply to the face. Massage well and leave for fifteen minutes. Remove with a damp facecloth and rinse thoroughly.

Banana Wrinkle-Fighter

(TO TIGHTEN SKIN AND REDUCE FINE LINES)

Mash half a banana and spread over the face, leaving for up to twenty minutes. Rinse away with lukewarm water.

Baking-Soda Toner

(TO WAKE UP THOSE PORES)

Make up a paste of around three parts baking soda (bicarbonate of soda) to one part water and rub onto a clean face. Rinse with lukewarm water.

Egg-White Toner

(TO CLEAN SKIN AND TIGHTEN PORES)

Smooth a raw egg white onto cleansed skin and leave for at least fifteen minutes. Wash off with warm water.

Strawberry and Banana Toner

(TO EXFOLIATE AND TIGHTEN SKIN)

Mash together a banana and a few ripe strawberries. Apply to the face and leave for fifteen minutes. Rinse away with clean warm water.

Cucumber Eye Tonic

(TO TIGHTEN UP THE SKIN UNDER THE EYES)

Grate cucumber and spread it under your eyes to tighten saggy skin and reduce the appearance of dark circles. Rinse with warm water after twenty minutes.

Lemon Teeth and Mouth Freshener

Rub the outer side of lemon peel over your teeth to remove stains such as tea, coffee or red wine. Make sure you rinse with water afterwards to prevent the acid in the lemon peel from damaging your enamel.

Lip Balm for Less

Smear Vaseline on your lips to protect them from extreme weather conditions and stop them getting chapped and dry – it works like a lipgloss too!

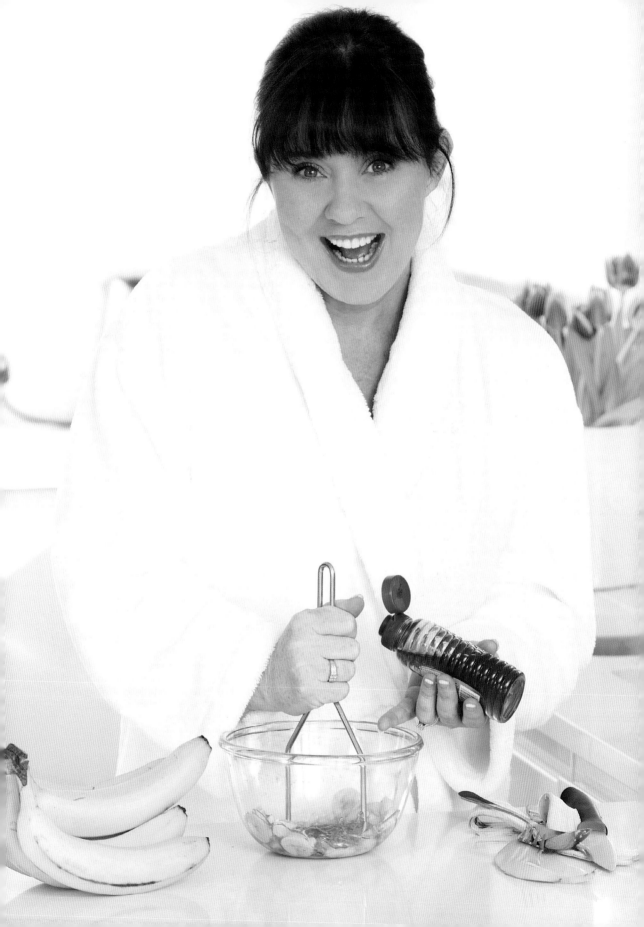

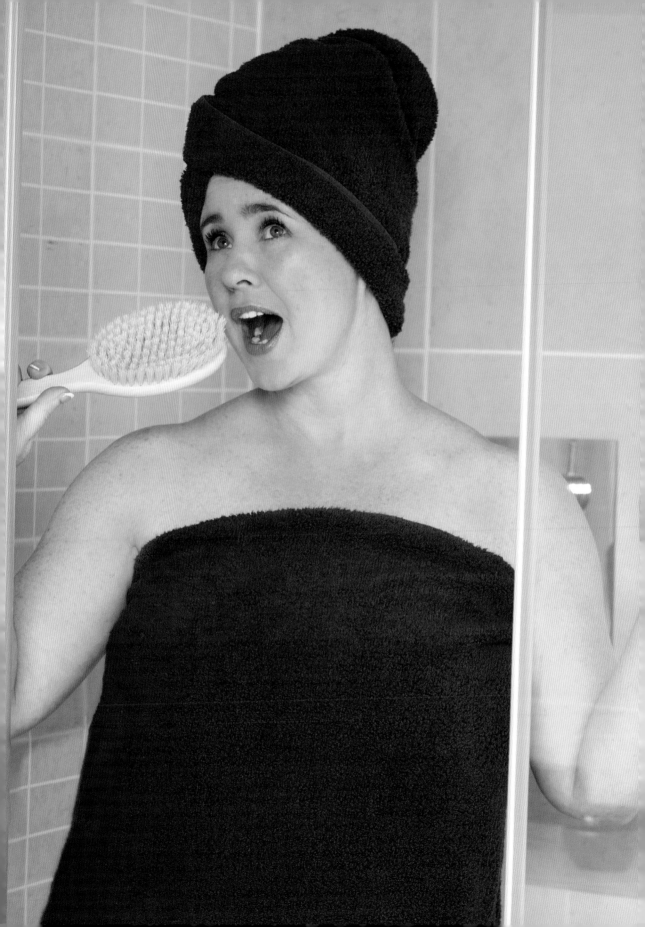

CHAPTER 3

*Spirit, body
and soul...*

YOUR BODY

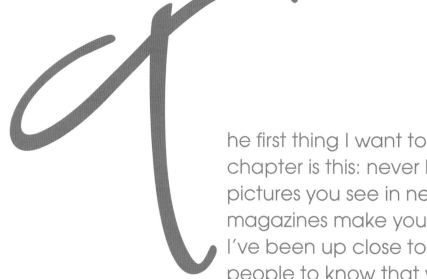

he first thing I want to say in this chapter is this: never let the celebrity pictures you see in newspapers and magazines make you feel depressed. I've been up close to enough famous people to know that what you see in the glossies is often not the real story.

The celebrities have usually been helped by expert lighting, professional styling and heavy make-up. And it's amazing what they can do with a picture these days: elongate the legs, airbrush out the cellulite, carry out a tummy tuck – and all with just one click of the computer mouse.

I'm not saying this is wrong – it's just another form of entertainment after all – but you can't necessarily believe what you see. Everyone knows, for example, that *Coronation Street* is just a work of fiction; you can't really go into the Rovers and order Betty's hotpot!

I was so worried about women comparing themselves with these images that I agreed to do some pictures with my *Loose Women* colleagues Denise Welch and Andrea McLean, on the promise that the photographs would be completely untouched. I wanted to show what the bodies of real women look like in their thirties (Andrea), forties (me) and fifties (Denise).

'BE HAPPIER WITH YOUR OWN BODY… AND LEARN TO MAKE THE MOST OF IT'

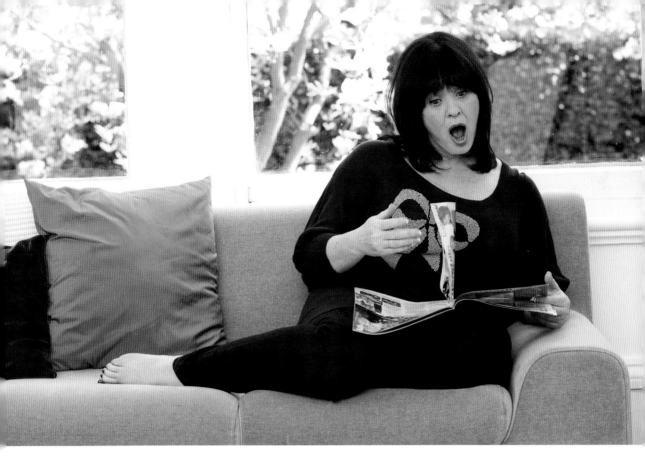

You see, in the past I've been the woman sitting at home in my tracksuit, hiding myself away. And when you're fed up with the way you look, airbrushed pictures make you feel like a different species to the women you see in magazines.

So, **LESSON ONE:** don't believe all that you see and start yearning for the unobtainable. And **LESSON TWO:** be happier with your own body…and learn to make the most of it. Having soft, smooth skin will certainly boost your body confidence and if you feel amazing underneath your clothes, it will shine through.

Most of us wouldn't dream of leaving the house without clean, conditioned hair and popping on a bit of lipstick, so why neglect the rest? Why is it that we spend 90 per cent of our time obsessing about the 10 per cent of us that's on show?

Smooth, silky, gloriously fragranced skin can be as exciting and effective a confidence boost as a designer dress, as well as being much cheaper. Tell yourself that you deserve a few moments to look after the 90 per cent – and what's more it doesn't have to take hours or cost a fortune.

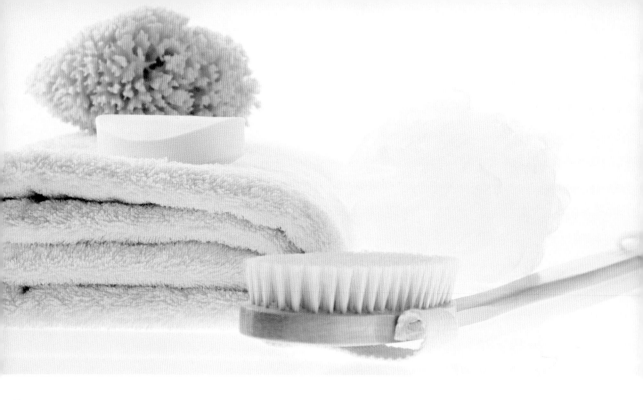

PERFECT SKIN

HOPEFULLY BY NOW YOU WILL BE IN A NEW ROUTINE THAT INVOLVES TAKING EXPERT CARE OF THE SKIN ON YOUR FACE. NOW IT'S TIME TO THINK ABOUT THE SKIN ON THE REST OF YOUR BODY. HERE'S A PLAN TO BOOST YOUR BODY CONFIDENCE:

Step One: Dry Brushing

Just as your face benefits from exfoliation, so will your body. Exfoliating shower gels are good, but even better is a regular rub down with a soft, dry brush before showering.

The experts say that dry brushing will take away the body's dead skin, tone muscles, stimulate circulation, reduce cellulite, prevent dry skin and eliminate toxins, therefore decreasing puffiness and swelling. Phew! And on top of all that it will also leave you feeling invigorated and ready for the day.

Use a soft brush with a long handle so that you can reach everywhere. A dry loofah or rough towel can work just as well. It doesn't matter where you start, but always stroke towards your heart so you don't put too much pressure on your circulatory system. Go easier on thinner skin, too, but brush away with gusto where the skin is thicker, such as on the soles of your feet. You should also avoid sensitive areas, such as the nipples, and any broken skin.

If you've got plenty of time, then fifteen minutes' dry brushing every day will work wonders. But back in the real world, do it as often and for as long as you can manage and you'll still see a difference. I've got it down to about five minutes now.

Step Two: Cleansing

Remember those scenes in *Carry on Cleo* where Cleopatra lounges around in her huge bath of milk and rose petals? I dream of moments like that. Instead of which, I have to fight three kids and a husband just to get into the bathroom. I'm lucky if I can grab five minutes' peace in the shower. I make sure I've always got a nice shower gel on the go or, if I'm doing really well, gorgeous bath bubbles to help me soak away the day.

HERE'S MY RUNDOWN OF WHAT'S ON THE MARKET:

● *Bar Soap*

There's nothing wrong with using the family bar of soap, but it can leave your skin feeling dry. Keep it for hand-washing and instead choose a simple, non-perfumed bar that will leave your skin feeling clean but not tight.

● *Body Wash*

Handy if a shower's all you have time for. Many body washes have moisturising ingredients in them, so they'll get you clean and leave your skin feeling soft.

● *Bubble Bath*

Check the ingredients for a moisturiser in your bubble bath if you don't want to leave the water feeling less hydrated than when you went in. You can always add a drop of almond or baby oil to the water to leave you feeling silky smooth.

● *Body Scrub*

Even if you dry-brush regularly, it's good to give your body an exfoliating session every now and then. Body scrubs have tiny synthetic beads or natural grains in them that remove dead skin cells and leave you feeling refreshed. A facecloth that can be chucked in the laundry is good for this, too, rather than a loofah kept in the shower, which can be a breeding ground for bacteria. Check to see if your body scrub includes a cleanser, otherwise you'll need soap as well. Concentrate on your elbows, knees, shins and the tops of your arms, and go lightly on sensitive areas.

● *Bath Bombs, Oils and Salts*

If you're lucky enough to have time for a good soak, then these are a real indulgence, although they won't get you clean. Take care not to mix too many fragrances. I steer clear of these bathroom treats if I'm going out later: I'd rather give off the scent of my favourite perfume than smell like a giant pineapple or coconut.

● *Sensitive-Skin Products*

If you're a sensitive type you'll know that many gels, scrubs and washes can be too harsh. Look out for hypo-allergenic, non-perfumed products that will be kinder to your skin.

Step Three: Moisturising

I admit it, when I was younger life was too short for body lotion. But as our skin becomes a little more…ahem…mature, you can almost hear it screaming out, 'Moisturise me!' Now I can't have a bath or shower without moisturising afterwards; my body just feels too dry without it.

To slow down the body's ageing process – and to feel smooth and sexy under your clothes – you need to get into the habit of applying body lotion every time you bathe. Some experts will tell you to choose different creams for different parts of the body, but I think life's too short for that. Just remember to cover the areas most prone to dryness, such as the lower legs, thighs, arms, elbows and knees.

Choose a moisturiser that matches your skin type – dry, sensitive, mature – and don't be fooled into thinking that the more money you pay for it, the better it will be. I prefer a lighter lotion that sinks into my skin easily and doesn't feel greasy. For years I've used a very basic, inexpensive, non-perfumed brand that leaves my skin feeling soft and supple.

Apply all over your dry body just after you've had a bath or shower – the heat will have opened your pores and the moisturiser will be more easily absorbed.

If you're really in a hurry and don't have time to apply lotion, make sure you use a shower gel that contains a moisturiser, as that will be less drying than soap. Try to moisturise properly as often as possible, though. And even if you are in a huge rush, never feel tempted to use body moisturiser on your face. Go up as far as the top of your neck, but stop there: your face is far too sensitive for body lotion.

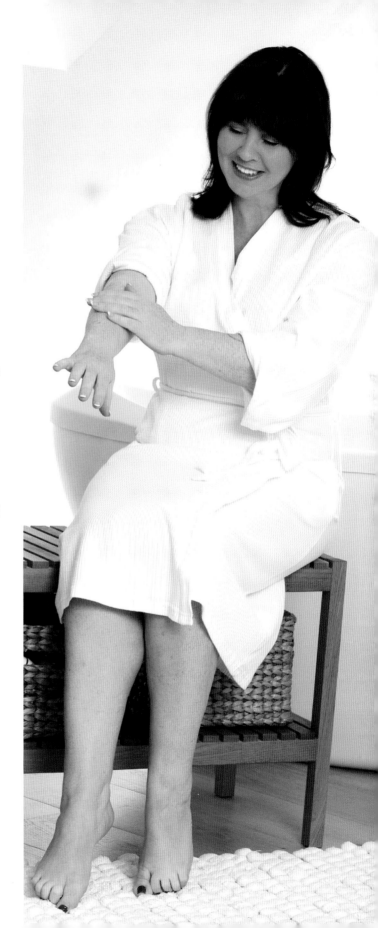

Create a Spa in Your Bathroom

Do you dream of being pampered in a beautiful spa? Of relaxing in wonderful surroundings? Of having the stresses of your day lifted from your shoulders by soothing music, flickering candles and scent so heavenly it carries you off into blissful sleep? You do? Then what's stopping you? Oh yes, I'd forgotten about the kids, the washing, work and a hole in your bank balance where oodles of spare cash should be.

But fear not, there is a way you can have your wish without it costing you a fortune. All you need are a few items that should be lying around the house, your bathroom and some precious time – that might be the tricky bit, but give it a go, then follow these ten steps to heaven.

MY TEN STEPS TO HEAVEN:

1 The night before your spa experience give your bathroom a thorough clean and get the enamel sparkling. You won't relax if you can see the taps need polishing. Throw your robe and favourite towels in the washing machine and get them dried, aired and really fluffy, ready for the big day – you wouldn't find coffee stains on your robe and torn-up hankies in your pocket at a top spa, would you?

2 Negotiate some time for yourself. You'll relax more in an empty house, but if this isn't possible, make sure you're not the one looking after the kids and make a 'DO NOT DISTURB' sign to hang on your bathroom door. Turn off your phone.

3 Make sure your bathroom is nice and warm, reduce the lighting and place some flowers from the garden and some lit scented candles safely around the room. Take your iPod dock or radio in with you and tune it to some relaxing music.

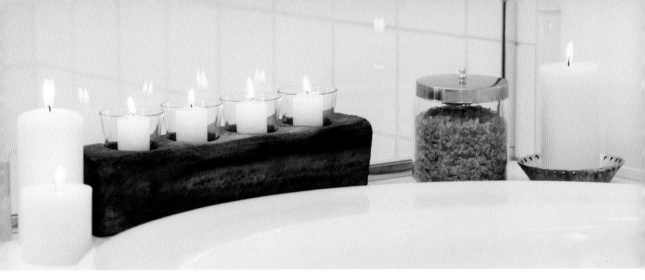

4 Include in your spa kit some chilled water in a bottle and that good book you've been desperate to read.

5 Run a warm bath and pour in some lovely bath oils or bubbles. Roll a fluffy towel into a headrest and step in, laying your head on the towel.

6 Spend as much time as you like relaxing, reading, listening to the music and thinking how lucky you are. Remember to keep sipping the drinking water.

7 Use the time to give your hair a deep condition, apply a face mask or use a scrub to exfoliate your body (you could use one of the home-made recipes at the end of this chapter).

8 When you're ready (or when the rest of the household can stand it no longer) step slowly from your bath and pat yourself dry with the warm fluffy towels.

9 Moisturise your skin while the temperature of your body is still raised.

10 Think to yourself that you deserve a little pampering every now and then and book another DIY spa session soon.

CELLULITE

IS THERE A SINGLE WOMAN WHO DOESN'T HAVE CELLULITE? I KNOW I SAID NOT TO BELIEVE WHAT YOU SEE IN MAGAZINES, BUT I MAKE AN EXCEPTION WHEN THE PICTURES EXPOSE A SUPERMODEL'S ORANGE-PEEL SKIN – THAT MAKES ME FEEL MUCH BETTER!

Cellulite is the collection of fat underneath the skin that can give our bums, thighs and underarms a dimpled, quilted appearance. Squeeze together the skin on your thighs to see if you've got it (although I'm sure you won't need me to point it out) – you're very lucky if you haven't. Although cellulite is linked to fat levels, you see it even on skinny women and it's almost impossible to get rid of.

I have to admit cellulite isn't one of my bigger worries. I'm sure I've got it lurking around the back of my thighs, but I'm too concerned about the front bits to worry about that. If I can't see it, why stress?

IF YOU'RE TROUBLED BY IT, HOWEVER, THERE ARE SOME STEPS YOU CAN TRY AS A DETERRENT:

- *Exercise*
Even gentle exercise such as swimming, brisk walking or cycling can help replace fat with muscle and improve your skin's appearance.

- *Massage*
It doesn't have to cost you a fortune; you can do it yourself. Apply a moisturising oil or lotion, then clench your fists and move them in circles firmly on your thighs and buttocks – you might want to ask your partner to help!

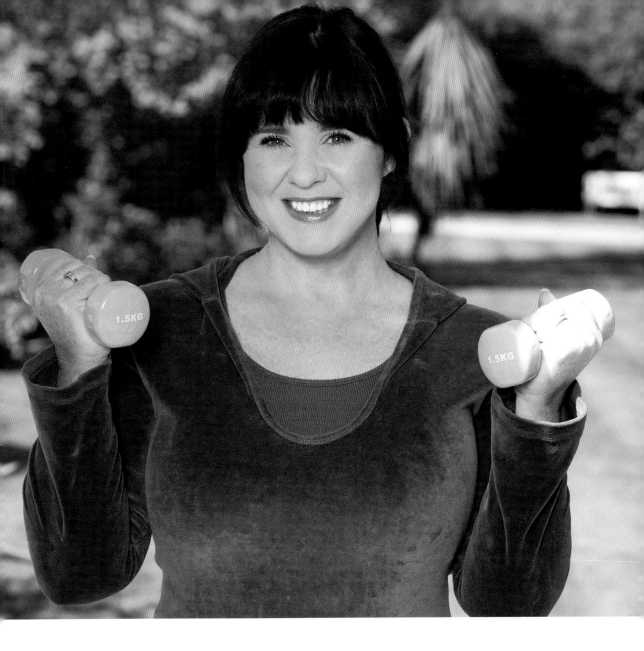

● *Water Jets*

Another DIY treatment. Turn your power shower on to its highest setting and blast your orange-peel areas.

● *Eat and Drink Well*

Cut down on processed foods and reduce your fat intake, replacing butter and cheese with low-fat alternatives. Make sure you drink at least eight glasses of water a day.

A CLOSE SHAVE

I LOVE BEING A BRUNETTE AND THESE DAYS WOULD NEVER THINK ABOUT GOING BLONDE, BUT ONE CONSEQUENCE OF BEING DARK IS THE CONSTANT BATTLE WITH UNWANTED HAIR – ON MY BODY AND ON MY FACE. IT'S A PAIN, ISN'T IT? NO SOONER HAVE I GOT RID OF IT THAN IT'S BACK AGAIN.

For example, as I've got older I've grown these three hairs on my chin – I'm turning into Billy Goat Gruff! I remember my *Loose Women* colleague Carol McGiffin once pulling at what she thought was a long stray hair on my face – you should have heard the shrieks when she realised it was still attached to my chin!

In the winter it's tempting to cover up in trousers and long sleeves and not even think about the areas we're supposed to keep tidy, but in this new era of becoming a beauty goddess, perhaps it's time to find a fast, cheap and painless way to be fuzz-free.

For years I only ever used a trusty razor and gave my legs and armpits a quick once-over every time I went in the bath. Then, when I lost weight and started doing swimwear shoots, I realised I was going to have to extend the operation and tackle my bikini line.

Some women take hair removal extremely seriously and go to lengths that would make your eyes water – literally! These days it's seen as trendy to have bikini-line waxes that remove almost everything, but busy mums may think this a beauty routine too far, and I must admit it's only ever a short back and sides for me.

There are good reasons to stay fuzz-free under your arms and on your legs. Hairless armpits feel cleaner and deodorants work more effectively when applied directly to the skin, while hairless legs give you a smoother line, even under tights, and a slimmer silhouette.

Shaving

Fast and cheap, this is the option I usually go for. It's suitable for underarms, legs and the bikini line and regrowth will start within a day or two. You can always nick your partner's razor blades, though don't say I said so as they *really* hate this. Make sure you shave when the hair is wet so the skin is soft, and use a shaving foam or gel to keep the skin moisturised – again, you can pinch his stuff but women's shaving products will smell nicer.

Did you know that if you run out of shaving foam, hair conditioner works just as well? Also, regular exfoliation and moisturising – we're doing that now, right? – will help prevent ingrowing hairs.

Electric Shaving

There's obviously the initial cost of the razor to be taken into consideration, although you'll never need to buy razor blades or shaving foam again. Electric razors won't nick you or dry out your skin so much, but the shave they give is rarely as close. There are some electric razors on the market that are waterproof and can be used in the shower or bath, but read the instructions carefully.

Epilator

An epilator grabs hairs in its revolving rollers and pulls them out at the roots. Oh my goodness it was painful the first time I tried it. I had to stuff my free fist in my mouth to stop myself screaming. On the plus side, epilators are fast and will leave you fuzz-free for about a month. And the good news is that the next time will be much less painful and the hairs that grow back will be finer and easier to remove. I have friends who use an epilator for all their hairy bits, but it's a little too painful for me in the more sensitive areas. Just like the electric shaver, there is the initial cost of the epilator, but it should last for years.

Depilatory Creams

You'll find a mind-boggling array of these products in the shops, some more expensive than others, but they all do the same basic job. They remove fuzz from the surface of the skin by dissolving the hair, which is then washed away. I used to hate the smell but they've improved over the years. They're suitable for armpits, legs and bikini lines, but if you want to use a depilatory cream down below, make sure it's a specially formulated one for sensitive areas.

Waxing

This is for the real – and brave – beauty goddess and will generally cost you more than shaving or hair-removal creams. You can wax at home or at a salon, but the basic process is the same: a sticky wax is applied to the hairy area, a strip is put on top and then pulled off quickly, ripping the hair out at the root. It can leave you hair-free for up to six weeks and regrowth will be finer. Waxing is suitable for all areas but the hair should be at least a quarter of an inch long. Some women – and men, amazingly – visit salons to have their nether regions waxed; it's painful but very quick and is perhaps better for those hard-to-reach areas. You may have heard of a Brazilian, where everything down under is whipped off, except for a thin 'landing strip' in the middle; but did you know that the Full Monty means having it all taken away? Ouch!

Permanent Hair Removal

If you really suffer from excessive body hair, you might want to seek advice on electrolysis or laser treatments. Electrolysis and laser hair removal are the only treatments that claim to permanently rid you of body hair. Both are expensive – we're talking at least £5 for five minutes of professional treatment and you will need a lot of sessions of around twenty minutes a go. Perhaps, though, this is something worth considering if you really hate having to keep your skin fuzz-free. They can also be very effective for women with facial-hair problems.

Electrolysis involves inserting a very fine needle into the base of the hair follicle and zapping it with an electric current to damage the root and stop it producing hair. It can take a year of regular treatments and is said to be quite painful, but the experts reckon it is most likely to result in a permanent solution.

Laser treatments are less painful because the beam of light that is used to damage the hair follicle attacks hundreds of roots at a time. Fewer treatments are needed but the jury still seems to be out on whether it is as effective as electrolysis – you might need more sessions every few months to top up the treatment, which can obviously work out expensive.

I've noticed you can buy DIY versions of both machines for around the same price as an epilator but the small print recommends you only use in limited areas, such as the face or arms. Treatments on larger body areas are usually done in beauty salons by specialists.

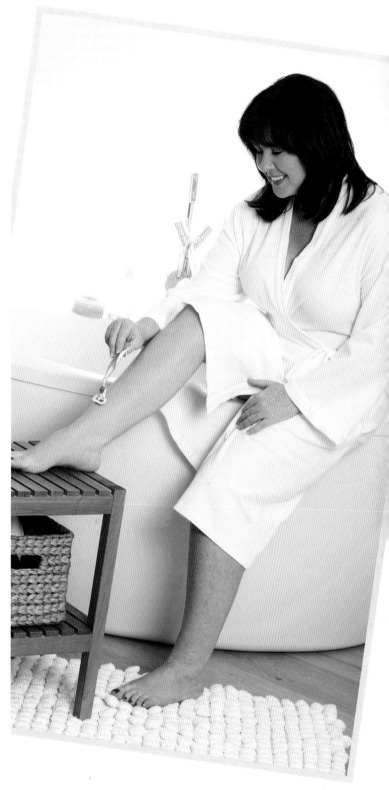

HERE COMES THE SUN

PEOPLE SAY THAT A GOLDEN TAN MAKES YOU FEEL FANTASTIC, THOUGH WITH MY PALE COMPLEXION IT'S NOT SOMETHING I'VE GOT MUCH EXPERIENCE OF. I TURN LOBSTER RED AND THEN MY SKIN PEELS OFF IF THE SUN SO MUCH AS WINKS AT ME.

Tanned skin can also make you look slimmer, so I understand why people are tempted to spread out on a sunbed the minute their holidays start. These days, knowing what we know about the dangers of skin cancer, it's just not OK to get burned. And while it's really important to cover up the kids – Ciara is used to me chasing her with factor 35 the moment the sun pops out – it's equally important to care for your own skin, too.

We've already talked about the importance of using an SPF moisturiser or make-up on your face. But you should also get used to slapping it on your body – just think about how many hours your hands and chest spend in the sunshine. These areas are most at risk from the harmful rays of the sun, and they're also the bits that start to wrinkle and age first.

When you're in the sun – not just on holiday but at home during the summer months – get used to using a body lotion that contains an SPF. The higher the SPF, the better the protection. But remember to use a proper sun cream with a higher SPF if you're whipping your clothes off and spending time in the hot sun. This isn't just a health warning, it's a beauty alert, too. If you want younger-looking, smooth skin, don't fry it to a crisp in the sunshine.

For most people, there's the option of using one of the many self-tanning lotions on the market. They can turn you every shade from a light glow to a deep tan, but remember you'll still need sunscreen. Alternatively you could treat yourself to a salon fake tan

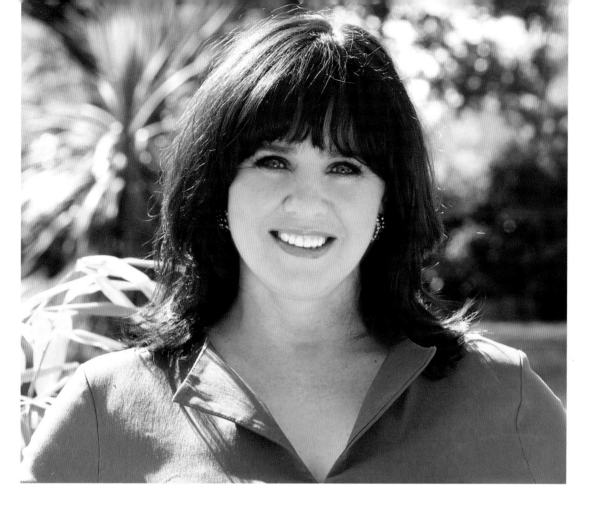

before your hols, but go easy: only *Strictly Come Dancing* contestants can get away with looking like a tangerine.

Unfortunately I'm really allergic to any form of fake tan; there's a chemical in them that does dreadful things to me. I only discovered this in 2007, the second time I tried using one. I'd had a spray tan for my wedding and felt fantastic, but the next time I tried it, a few months later, I came out in a terrible rash. Then when I went on *Dancing on Ice* the wardrobe people tried a new kind of fake tan on me. I had it on the Friday and by Sunday hives were creeping up my neck – I ended up bathed in calamine lotion. After that, you might remember, my costumes always covered my chest and arms, so I didn't look paler than everyone else.

These days I either have to put up with looking like a milk bottle or try to get a natural look using bronzing powder. When we're on holiday I always cover up with a hat and a T-shirt – no more sunburn or fake tans for me; they're just not worth the misery.

MAKING SCENTS

ONE OF MY EARLIEST MEMORIES IS OF PUTTING MY NOSE IN MY MUM'S WARDROBE AND BREATHING IN THE PERFUME ON HER CLOTHES.

I think it was an Estée Lauder perfume and I can still smell it now. I'd sit at her dressing table and dab it on my wrists and neck, just like I'd seen her do. When I was old enough to have my own perfume, I'd line up the bottles and spray enough on me each morning to last the whole week. I can still remember them: Anaïs Anaïs, Maxi and Charlie. I loved perfume then and I love it now – I think every woman should have a signature scent, or even a few of them. My favourites are Calvin Klein's Euphoria and J'adore by Dior. When I go away I spray Ciara's teddy bear with my perfume; that way if she's missing me she can still feel close to me.

Perfume doesn't have to be ridiculously expensive; just choose one that makes you feel lovely. It's also the perfect birthday or Christmas gift. Next time you're passing a perfume counter, try sniffing a few new ones to see what takes your fancy.

• Did You Know...

Eau de cologne, or eau fraîche as it's sometimes known, is the lightest scent with the least perfume concentrate, and will only stay fragrant for about an hour.

Eau de toilette has slightly more perfume in it and will cost a little more but is still affordable. You'll smell gorgeous for a few hours.

Eau de parfum is the biggest selling type of perfume and should stay fragrant for most of the day.

Perfume is the most concentrated and most expensive but should last all day.

Tip: *Make your perfume last longer by keeping it in the fridge. It needs a little warmth to bring out the full fragrance. That's why it's dabbed on the neck and wrists – pulse points get perfume cooking nicely.*

Finding the Fragrance for You

Perfumes fall into one of several groups that suit particular types of women, or so the experts reckon. I say, just have a sniff and choose the one you like (or can afford). You might want to ask a friend to give you her honest opinion, though, as perfume is a funny thing and what you smell isn't necessarily what others smell too.

➡ **FLORAL:** *contains hints of flowers such as rose, jasmine and gardenias and suits most age groups.*
Typical floral perfume: *Beautiful by Estée Lauder.*

➡ **CITRUS:** *packed with lemon, lime or tangerine, this fragrance is supposed to suit younger women, but if you like it, go for it.*
Typical citrus perfume: *CK One by Calvin Klein.*

➡ **WOODY:** *scents of sandalwood and cedar are to be found in this perfume. Supposedly one for more mature ladies.*
Typical woody perfume: *Coco Mademoiselle by Chanel.*

➡ **ORIENTAL:** *muskier fragrance, with hints of spices. This is quite a sophisticated perfume and not necessarily suited to younger women.*
Typical oriental perfume: *Opium by Yves St Laurent.*

➡ **GREEN:** *this type of perfume is said to be fresh and remind you of being outdoors. Good for younger, sportier women.*
Typical green perfume: *Charlie by Revlon (yes, it's still here after all these years!).*

HELP YOURSELF FOR FREE

I LOVE BEING GIVEN YUMMY BODY WASHES AND RELAXING BUBBLE BATH FOR BIRTHDAYS AND CHRISTMAS, EVEN THOUGH I HAVE TO HIDE THEM AWAY FROM THE REST OF THE HOUSEHOLD. IN AN IDEAL WORLD I'D HAVE A NEVER-ENDING SUPPLY, BUT THEY CAN BE EXPENSIVE. HERE'S HOW YOU CAN ALWAYS HAVE SOME TO HAND WITHOUT BREAKING THE BANK.

- ### Cleo's Bath
Tip two cups of powdered or fresh milk into a warm bath for lovely soft skin.

- ### Chocoholic's Bath
Mix two cups of powdered milk with a quarter of a cup of cocoa and two tablespoons of cornflour. Add to a warm bath for a delicious treat.

- ### Coffee Scrub
The next time you make a cup of fresh coffee, save the grounds and mix three tablespoons with one tablespoon of coarse salt. Rub the mixture over your body while you're in the shower, then rinse with warm water and moisturise.

- ### Cinna-Bath
Mix a quarter of a cup of powdered milk with a quarter of a cup of baking powder, half a tablespoon of cornflour and half a tablespoon of cinnamon. Tip into hot running water for a delicious smelling, relaxing bath.

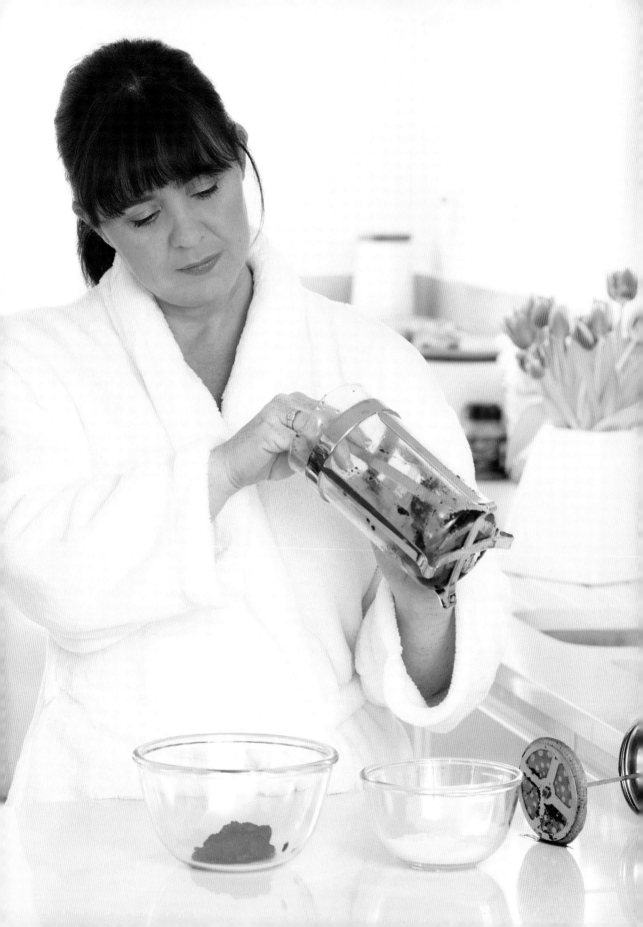

Honey and Vanilla Bubbles

Mix a cup of olive oil with half a cup of mild liquid soap and a quarter of a cup of honey. Add a few drops of vanilla extract, put in a bottle and shake to mix well. Shake the bottle each time you use it and pour under hot running water for a bubbly bath.

Lavender and Milk Bath

Mix half a cup of powdered milk with two tablespoons of dried lavender and tip into hot running water. Feel the stresses of your day disappear.

Ginger and Cinammon Bath Scrub

Mix one cup of sea salt with half a teaspoon each of ground ginger and ground cinammon. Add a cup of olive oil and rub over your skin. Relax into a warm bath and rinse. This will improve your circulation and make you feel energised.

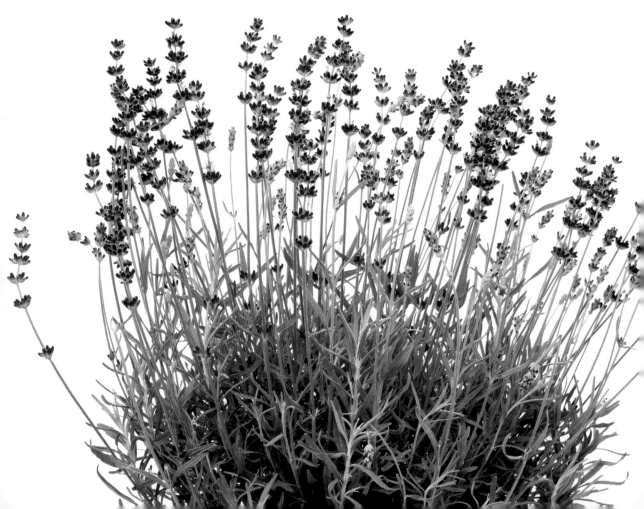

Sugar Scrub

Mix a cup of brown or white sugar with half a cup of olive oil and a few drops of perfumed oil. Rub it all over your body while you're in the bath for a sweet exfoliation. Rinse with warm water, dry your body and moisturise.

Fresh Sea Scrub

For a fresh scrub, use two parts coarse sea salt to one part Epsom salts (available from your chemist) and mix with a few drops of mild liquid soap and some drops of perfumed oil if you wish. Scrub all over your body, then rinse and moisturise.

Make Your Own Bath Bomb

This is a little trickier than the bath soaks and scrubs, but it's fun to do and would save those who like a fizz in their bath a lot of money.

FOLLOW THIS RECIPE FOR A BASIC BOMB:

1. *5 teaspoons of olive oil*
2. *1½ cups of bicarbonate of soda*
3. *½ a cup of citric acid (can be bought in a brewer's shop or chemist)*
4. *10 drops of perfumed oil*
5. *A few drops of food colouring*
6. *Water to mix*

Add the olive oil to the bicarbonate of soda and citric acid, stir, and add the perfume and food colouring, then slowly add a tablespoon of water, drop by drop (any faster and the bomb will fizz too early). Use your hands to shape the mixture into balls – if it's too dry, add extra water – making it as smooth as possible. Leave until it's dried out completely. Makes around six fizzy bath bombs.

Bath-Bomb Sparkler

Mix half a teaspoon of glitter to the dry ingredients for a magical bath.

Wake-Up Bath Bomb

Follow the basic bath-bomb recipe, but add a few drops of lemon essential oil instead of perfumed oil. This is sure to get you going!

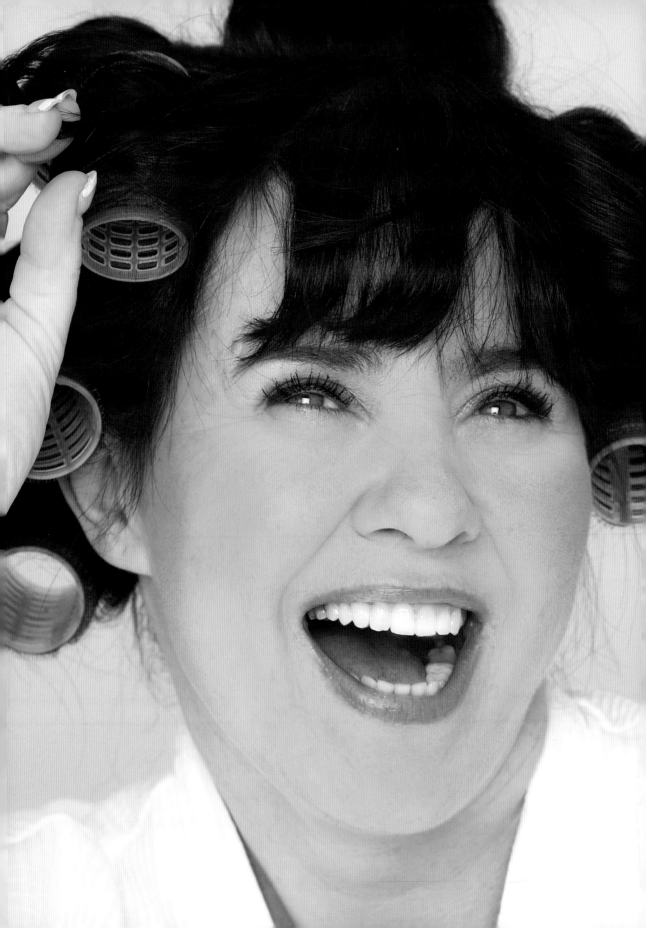

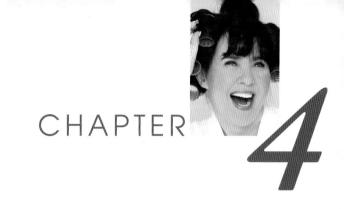
Don't make waves…

YOUR HAIR

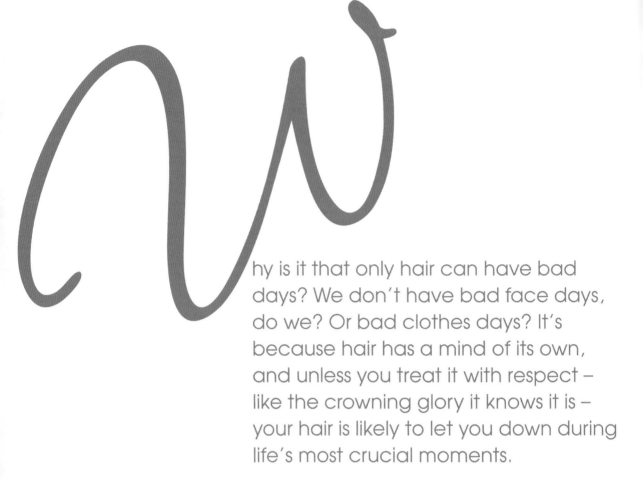

Why is it that only hair can have bad days? We don't have bad face days, do we? Or bad clothes days? It's because hair has a mind of its own, and unless you treat it with respect – like the crowning glory it knows it is – your hair is likely to let you down during life's most crucial moments.

Well-conditioned, shiny hair that's been beautifully cut and nicely coloured will carry you through those days when you can't be bothered to make much of an effort in other areas. But if you neglect your locks, it won't matter how well you dress or make up your face, you'll still look like you've been dragged through a hedge backwards.

I now try not to mess with my hair too much, although there's one awful photograph that shows this wasn't always the case. I'm aged about sixteen and I have a poodle on my head. I'm not joking. Someone claiming to be a hairdresser has given me the world's worst perm and I am the spitting image of Kevin Keegan. I can still remember the day it happened. It was pouring with rain outside afterwards and I refused the salon's offer of an umbrella,

'I TRY NOT TO MESS WITH MY HAIR TOO MUCH'

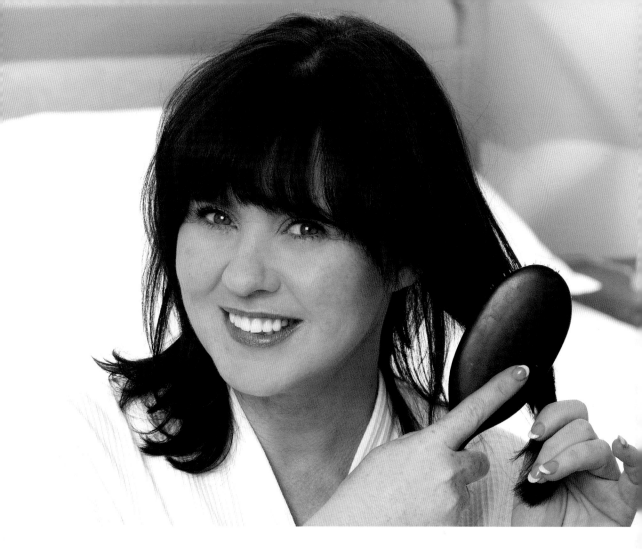

probably hoping that the rain would straighten it out. Of course it just made the curls even tighter and I sobbed as I ran home to our house.

The perm wasn't my only hair disaster in my youth. For most of my childhood I looked like a little boy because my dad used to cut my hair and would give me a short back and sides. Later on, as a teenager, I dyed my hair every colour imaginable: red, plum, even blonde. I remember walking into our house in Blackpool with a head full of thick, blonde highlights and Mum going berserk. She said it looked more grey than blonde and I must admit it made me look ten years older.

Since then I've generally kept my hair straight and dark. I've treated it kindly and now it's repaying me. People compliment me on my shiny, healthy hair, and if I am managing to keep one step ahead of the ageing process, I think it's partly thanks to that.

My husband, Ray, always notices my hair. He loves it straight and long and he hates it when I get adventurous. Sometimes I ask the *Loose Women* stylist to give me curls or to pin it up, but when I get home I can tell right away that he doesn't like it. Mind you, at least he notices!

I don't really suffer from hair envy, but if I could swap my locks with anyone else's I reckon it would be Angelina Jolie. Long, black and luscious, her hair always looks great. Jennifer Aniston also has beautiful hair. Maybe that's what first attracted Brad to both of them.

If you look at pictures of Ange and Jen, it's true to say that neither have fiddled much with their hair. It's basically the same long, well-conditioned style they've had for years. Which totally goes against the next thing I'm about to say...move with the times.

It's vital that you don't get stuck in a rut, unless of course you look like Mrs Pitt I or Mrs Pitt II, in which case feel free to do what you like! How often do you see a middle-aged woman who obviously found her style back in the Seventies or Eighties but still clings stubbornly to it? Just like make-up, a hairstyle that's obviously 'of its day' can age you terribly. So move with the times and don't stick with the same style all your life.

You can also experiment with colour. I've played with low lights and subtle changes, and as we get older it's important to cover up the inevitable grey (although it hasn't done George Clooney any harm – how unfair is that?).

A good hairdresser can advise on cut and colour and should become your friend and confidante. You shouldn't have to save up two weeks' wages in order to afford a ridiculously expensive salon. Just ask around and try different people until you find a hairdresser you feel comfortable with. The right person will be honest with you, won't make you feel intimidated and when they ask you if you're going anywhere nice on holiday, they'll genuinely want to know.

You should also be brave and take in a photograph of the style you fancy. Unless you're in your dotage and requesting 'a Jennifer', you should feel relaxed enough to ask for your hairdresser's opinion. And incidentally, if you are knocking on ninety and planning a Jen, you don't need my advice...you are fabulous already!

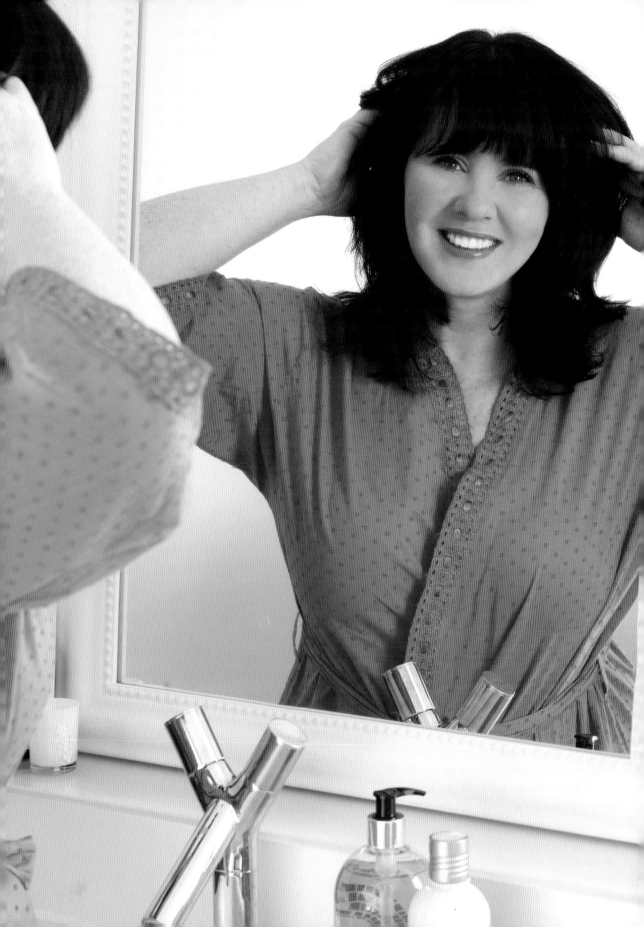

WHAT IS YOUR HAIR TYPE?

IN CHAPTER 1 WE USED THE TISSUE TEST TO DISCOVER OUR HAIR TYPE. DEPENDING ON THE AMOUNT OF OIL PRESENT ON THE SCALP YOUR HAIR WILL BE NORMAL, DRY OR GREASY. I WOULD SAY MY OWN HAIR IS NORMAL TO GREASY AND I HAVE TO WASH IT EVERY OTHER DAY. IF I GO ANY LONGER THAN THAT, IT FEELS DIRTY AND LOOKS REALLY LIMP.

IF YOU HAVE:

● Normal Hair

Your locks will naturally shine and shouldn't need washing more than two or three times a week. You still need to take care of your hair, though – don't take it for granted.

● Dry Hair

You find your hair damages easily, splitting at the ends and breaking when styled. It's never shiny and looks dull, even just after it's been washed and conditioned. You need to look at what's causing the damage. The chemicals you are putting on it? The heat you're inflicting on it? Is it down to your diet? Your lifestyle? The environment around you? You can buy specially formulated products that will enhance dry hair or try following these tips to end dry days for good:

- *Make sure you have a regular trim to get rid of split ends.*
- *The sun will dry out your hair, so on hot days use a special hair conditioner with an SPF or wear a hat.*
- *If you're a regular swimmer, the salt or chlorine in the water won't be doing your hair any favours. Wear a swimming cap – they can look quite glamorous, you know – and rinse your hair well after swimming.*
- *Don't shampoo your hair too often or you'll strip out all the good oils. If you really don't feel ready for the day without a hair wash, then just put shampoo on the roots and rinse away quickly.*
- *Take a breather from heated appliances. Go natural for a while and your hair will be grateful.*
- *Look after yourself. Eat a balanced diet, drink lots of water and make sure you have enough sleep.*
- *Try one of the conditioning treatments at the end of this chapter.*

Greasy Hair

Your locks can look good immediately after styling but quickly lose their body and bounce. Take care not to rub your head too briskly when you're washing your hair as that can stimulate the oil-producing glands on the scalp. Some experts say it's best not to wash greasy hair every day, but if you must, make sure you use a specially formulated shampoo for greasy hair, or an extremely gentle one. Follow these tips to say goodbye to the grease:

- *Use an oil-free shampoo and don't condition each time you wash. Use the conditioner only on the ends of the hair and not the roots.*
- *Make sure you rinse the shampoo out of your hair thoroughly.*
- *Try to touch your hair as little as possible – fingers, brushes and appliances will all help spread oil from the roots down the hair shaft.*
- *Clean your hairbrush and comb regularly so you don't spread grease back on to your freshly washed locks.*
- *Treat yourself to a newly washed pillowcase every night.*

When it comes to looking after your hair, always remember the three Cs: **CARE, CUT AND COLOUR**. Look after these three and you'll soon give Ange and Jen a run for their money.

HAIR CARE

IT SOUNDS OBVIOUS, BUT TO KEEP YOUR HAIR IN BEAUTIFUL CONDITION, YOU NEED TO KEEP IT CLEAN AND MOISTURISED, PROTECT IT FROM EXTREME TEMPERATURES AND CHEMICALS AND FEED IT FROM WITHIN.

Choose your shampoo and conditioner carefully, bearing your hair type in mind. There are hundreds of brands out there and you won't necessarily need to spend a fortune. Once you find the brand that's right for you, take the occasional holiday from it: you'll find the condition of your hair will improve when you start using it again. I use a separate conditioner on my hair every time I wash it, but I don't use a great deal of product each time.

Shampooing Tips

- Brush and detangle your hair before washing – this will stop it from getting knotty during the shampoo stage and prevent it from breaking.

- Make sure your hair is soaking wet before applying the shampoo, otherwise you won't be able to work up a good lather.

- Pour the shampoo onto your hand, not your head, and rub your palms together before smoothing it onto your scalp to ensure even coverage.

- Concentrate on the roots of your hair – the shampoo will spread everywhere else during the rinsing process.

- Use your fingertips, not your nails, to massage your scalp in circular motions.

- Don't believe the experts who tell you to rinse with ice-cold water – it's unnecessary and just horrible. Warm water, not hot, is perfect.

- Think you've rinsed enough? Then stay under that shower and rinse for five minutes more! Rinse your hair until it squeaks and it will be lovely and shiny.

- You will save money and stop a build-up of product on your hair by only doing one wash. I know the bottle says 'repeat', but that's just so you use it twice as fast.

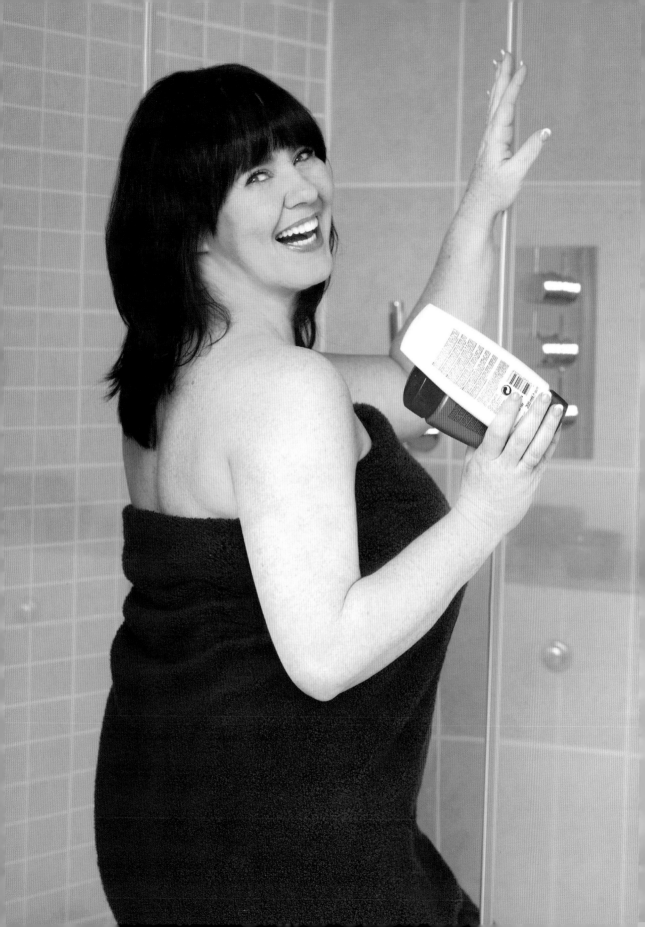

Emergency!

If you're really stuck for time, but desperate for clean hair, you could try one of the latest generation of dry shampoos. They sound like something from your mum's day, but apparently spray-on hair products are really taking off in these time-pressed times of ours.

All you do is spray the talc-based shampoo onto your hair, then brush through. They're supposed to clean and freshen your hair, soaking up the grease and giving you another day or so before you need to shampoo properly. Plus there's the added benefit of not needing to use a hairdryer or straightening irons on a daily basis. Just make sure you brush your hair thoroughly to remove all the talc, otherwise your locks could end up looking dull and grey.

Conditioning Tips

● After shampooing, squeeze the excess water from your hair as sopping-wet hair won't be able to absorb the conditioner. Even better, towel-dry your hair before applying conditioner, which will help your hair absorb it better.

● Squeeze a 50-pence-piece-sized blob of conditioner onto your hands and smooth your palms together.

● Starting at the hairline, work the conditioner through the hair, right to the ends – there's no need to massage conditioner into the roots of your hair.

● Use a wide-toothed comb to spread the conditioner right through the strands of your hair.

● Leave the conditioner on for a few minutes before rinsing well with warm water. Your hair should feel slippery when the conditioner is all rinsed away.

● Blot your hair with a towel; do not rub it or you'll end up with knots again. Wet hair is fragile, so use a clean comb to finish rather than a brush.

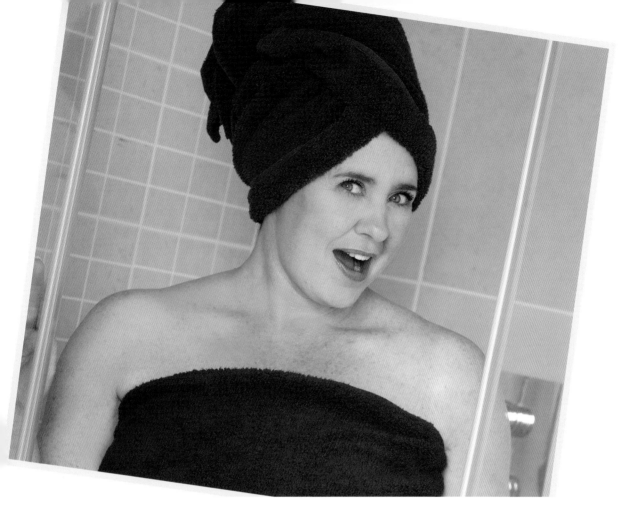

Extra Conditioning

There will be times when your hair needs a deeper conditioning treatment than usual. You might have messed it up with too many chemicals or spent too much time in the sun, but whatever the reason, it's time to call in the cavalry.

You'll find hair masks, hair tonics, deep conditioners and all manner of heavy-duty aids on the shelves of your chemist or supermarket. Most are expensive and some can be too harsh for your hair.

My advice would be to think first about prevention: protect your hair from heat and chemicals and you could save yourself time and money. Or you could buy a cheaper conditioning treatment and use it on a regular weekly basis. Alternatively, try one of my home-made recipes at the end of the chapter. It may feel strange sticking mayonnaise or a pint of beer on your bonce, but believe me it works.

THINNING HAIR

I KNOW FROM THE LETTERS I RECEIVE THAT THIS IS THE HAIR PROBLEM THAT WORRIES WOMEN MOST.

The experts say it's caused by hormonal changes, stress, illness, extreme dieting and lack of iron. Although most women find that their hair becomes wonderfully thick when they are pregnant, some suffer temporary hair loss, which thankfully tends to stop once the baby is born or soon after. I think my own hair is quite thin, but luckily I have a lot of it so it doesn't cause me too many problems.

Look for a shampoo and conditioner that gives you volume and eat plenty of iron-rich foods such as lean red meat or leafy green vegetables. Vitamin C helps the body absorb iron, so get your share of oranges, broccoli and kiwi fruit. You could also try massaging your scalp each day before washing your hair as this is said to improve circulation and stimulate hair growth. If you are very worried about hair loss, however, you should ask your doctor for advice.

DANDRUFF

IF YOU HAVE A PERSISTENTLY FLAKY, ITCHY SCALP, YOU COULD BE SUFFERING FROM A MEDICAL CONDITION SUCH AS ECZEMA OR PSORIASIS, SO ASK YOUR DOCTOR IF YOU'RE WORRIED. MY SCALP IS PRONE TO DRYNESS AND OCCASIONALLY I USE A MEDICATED SHAMPOO THAT HELPS MOISTURISE THE SKIN.

'ALWAYS RINSE YOUR HAIR THOROUGHLY AFTER WASHING SO AS NOT TO LET PRODUCTS BUILD UP'

Dandruff outbreaks are also thought to stem from a fungal infection of the skin so look out for anti-fungal shampoos, especially natural ones containing tea-tree oil.

You could also try dolloping some natural yoghurt on your head and letting it sit on the scalp for up to twenty-five minutes. Rinse and then wash with a mild shampoo before rinsing again thoroughly.

If you just have a dry, flaky scalp, try this olive oil treatment. Heat the oil by placing some in a small bowl inside a larger bowl containing hot water. Comb the oil through your hair, making sure your scalp is covered, then wrap your head in cling film for about twenty minutes. Shampoo as normal.

To make sure the white speckles falling onto your shoulders aren't left-in shampoo or hair products, always rinse your hair thoroughly after washing so as not to let hair products build up.

SPLIT ENDS

CHEMICALS AND HEAT CAN DAMAGE YOUR HAIR, CAUSING IT TO SPLIT AT THE ENDS.

The bad news is that the only cure is a visit to the hairdresser as they'll need to be snipped off. In the meantime, massage almond oil into the ends of your hair – you can do this on damp or dry hair – rubbing it in well so as to prevent further breakages until you can get to your hairdresser.

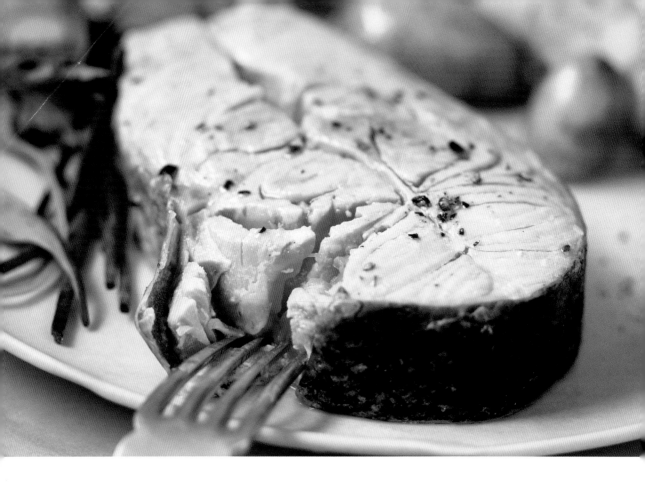

EATING WELL FOR LOVELY LOCKS

JUST AS OUR SKIN BENEFITS FROM A HEALTHY DIET, SO DOES OUR HAIR.
THINK OF YOURSELF AS A HEALTHY, HAPPY PET DOG WITH A SHINY COAT…
WELL, MAYBE NOT, BUT YOU GET THE IDEA.

If you've been on a crash diet you may have noticed that your hair has become dull and lifeless – proof that it needs properly balanced nutrition if it's to be shiny, bouncy and full of life.

The number one food for healthy hair is salmon, which is great because it's one of my favourite things. It's stuffed with Omega 3 fatty acids, which encourage hair growth. Dark green vegetables, eggs, whole grains, avocados, low-fat dairy products and nuts are all good for your hair, as are carrots, because they contain vitamin A, which helps nourish the scalp.

Remember that hair and nails are basically made of the same stuff, so what's good for your head is good for your hands. Eat a diet that's rich in vitamins, minerals, protein and Omega 3 and you will be gorgeous from head to toe.

Smooth as Silk

One final note on your hair's condition: try using a satin pillowcase if you want to have tresses like a princess.

Traditional cotton pillowcases are said to suck up the moisture from your hair, while satin or silk maintains it. Some experts say silky pillowcases also reduce knots and therefore breakages because your hair glides over the material. Satin sheets are thought to be better for your skin, too.

But before you rush out to update your linen cupboard, try a DIY trick and save your hard-earned cash. An old silk or satin shirt could easily be converted into a small pillowcase, or you could buy some material and get stitching.

CUT

REMEMBER BACK IN CHAPTER 1 I ASKED YOU TO TAKE A CLOSE LOOK AT THE SHAPE OF YOUR FACE? KNOWING WHETHER YOU HAVE AN OVAL, ROUND, SQUARE, LONG OR HEART-SHAPED FACE IS CRUCIAL WHEN IT COMES TO CHOOSING YOUR HAIRSTYLE.

With my oval-to-round face shape I have always been advised by hairdressers to go for a wispy fringe and keep the length long. There have been times over the years when I've longed for a cute pixie cut, but I know in my heart the stylists are right.

HERE ARE THE BEST STYLES FOR YOUR FACE SHAPE:

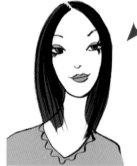

• Oval Face

A true oval is the face shape that suits most styles. Avoid very straight, dramatic fringes – opt for a layered fringe if you really want one – but apart from that feel free to experiment. Long, short, layered or curly, your face shape will look great whatever.

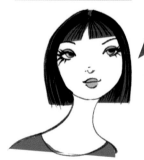

• Round Face

If this is you, you'll know it's best to go for styles that add volume. Short crops and snatched-back ponytails will emphasise your round cheeks and chin, so choose fuller styles with more body instead.

Square Face

For a more feminine look, soften your strong jaw line with layers around the face and steer clear of sharp bobs and straight fringes.

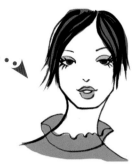

Long Face

Any style fringe will make your face look shorter, and you could emphasise the width of your face by going for a style that's full at the sides. A very short or very long style will only elongate your face more.

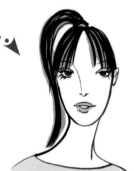

Heart-Shaped Face

Heart-shaped faces are wider at the forehead and pointier at the chin, so opt for a full fringe and add width at the sides. Shoulder-length hair in soft waves is the perfect look for you.

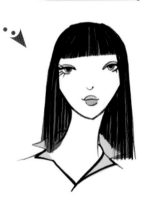

'WITH MY OVAL-TO-ROUND FACE SHAPE I HAVE ALWAYS BEEN ADVISED BY HAIRDRESSERS TO GO FOR A WISPY FRINGE AND KEEP THE LENGTH LONG. I KNOW IN MY HEART THE STYLISTS ARE RIGHT'

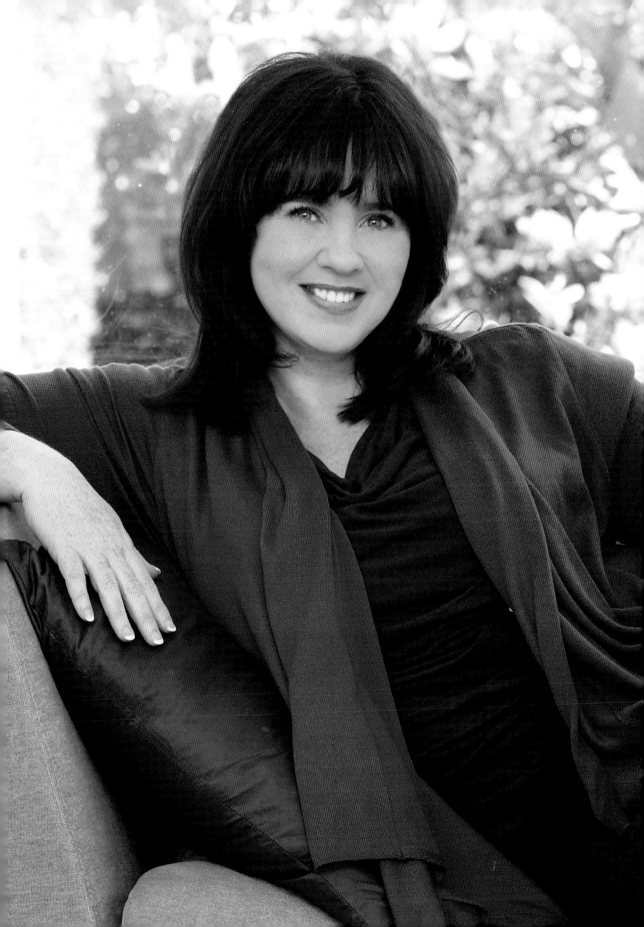

A GIRL'S BEST FRIEND

AS I SAID EARLIER IN THIS CHAPTER, YOU NEED TO BUILD A REALLY STRONG RELATIONSHIP WITH YOUR HAIRDRESSER. YOU MUST BE ABLE TO TRUST HIM OR HER AND BE ABLE TO ASK QUESTIONS, AND LIKEWISE THEY SHOULD KNOW YOUR PERSONALITY WELL ENOUGH TO MAKE SUGGESTIONS.

Don't ever be bullied into anything you're uncomfortable with and make sure you speak up when you're asked at the end what you think. Haircuts are an expensive business, so don't do what I did on the day I had my disaster perm and say, 'It's lovely,' then run home in tears.

Take with you a photograph from a celebrity or hair magazine so the stylist can see exactly what you're trying to achieve. I can remember doing this myself and I know at least two of my sisters cut out photographs of Pam Ewing from *Dallas* in the Seventies to get the look that was all the rage then.

Spend a good five or ten minutes with the stylist before you head off to get your hair washed – you both need to be very clear about what is about to happen. And be realistic. If the stylist says the texture of your hair will not suit the style you have chosen, ask them to suggest alternatives.

Once your hair is cut and the drying begins, watch the stylist closely to see how they blow-dry your hair. Ask for tips on technique and styling products, although beware, some hairdressers will try to flog you a bottle of expensive wonder gunk that you don't need.

COLOUR

SO, COLEEN, I HEAR YOU SAY, WHAT COLOUR IS YOUR HAIR NATURALLY? IT'S A SORT OF DULL, MOUSY BROWN AND IT'S BEEN A WHILE SINCE I LAST SAW IT, I MUST ADMIT.

I've never understood why anyone would want to stick with their own hair colour when there are so many better options out there. Adding colour to your hair can add brightness and depth as well as improving its condition. And if, like me, you've reached the age where grey hairs are starting their march for world domination, hair colour will also help you look younger.

Saying that, since those ill-fated highlights I've never been tempted to go blonde. With my pale complexion, fair hair makes me look slightly ill, so I've stuck to being a brunette, while waving goodbye to mousy years ago. The experts say you should stray no more than three shades from your natural colour and, unless your name is Pink and you have a pop career to pursue, this is probably excellent advice.

There are three main types of hair colourant: **highlights** (and **low lights**), **semi-permanent** and **permanent colour**.

Highlights and Low Lights

Narrow flashes of colour that compliment the rest of your hair. Highlights, usually in blonde colours, will brighten your look, whereas low lights, often in plum or auburn shades, will add depth. Highlights and low lights are usually permanent and should probably be done in a salon. It is possible to tackle this procedure yourself, but it's tricky, and mistakes could be disastrous.

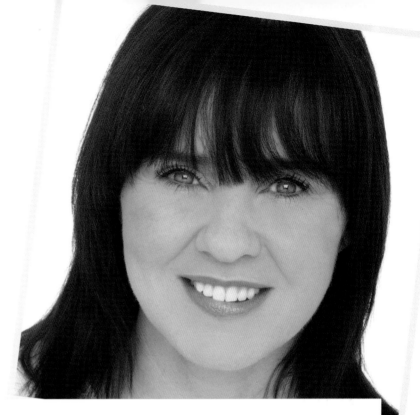

'YOU SHOULD STRAY NO MORE THAN THREE SHADES FROM YOUR NATURAL COLOUR'

Semi-Permanent Colour

This is what I use to cover the grey and give my hair depth and shine. A semi is an all-over hair colour that lasts for between six and eight weeks. It's gentler on your hair, but it can't change your colour dramatically and will struggle to make it lighter as it works by applying a layer of colour over the top of your existing shade. It will fade with each wash and won't leave you with noticeable roots. Semi-permanent colour is good for covering hair that is no more than 25 per cent grey and should leave your hair beautifully conditioned. It's fairly easy to do at home and won't damage your hair or leave you with irreversible mistakes.

Permanent Colour

If you want to dramatically change your hair colour, or if you have more than 25 per cent grey, then you'll need to use a permanent hair dye. These dyes contain peroxide and ammonia and work by stripping the pigment from your hair while depositing a new colour. Having your hair coloured at a salon is expensive and takes hours, so think about doing it yourself at home. The results are irreversible, though, so follow the instructions on the box carefully. If you do, you could achieve excellent results.

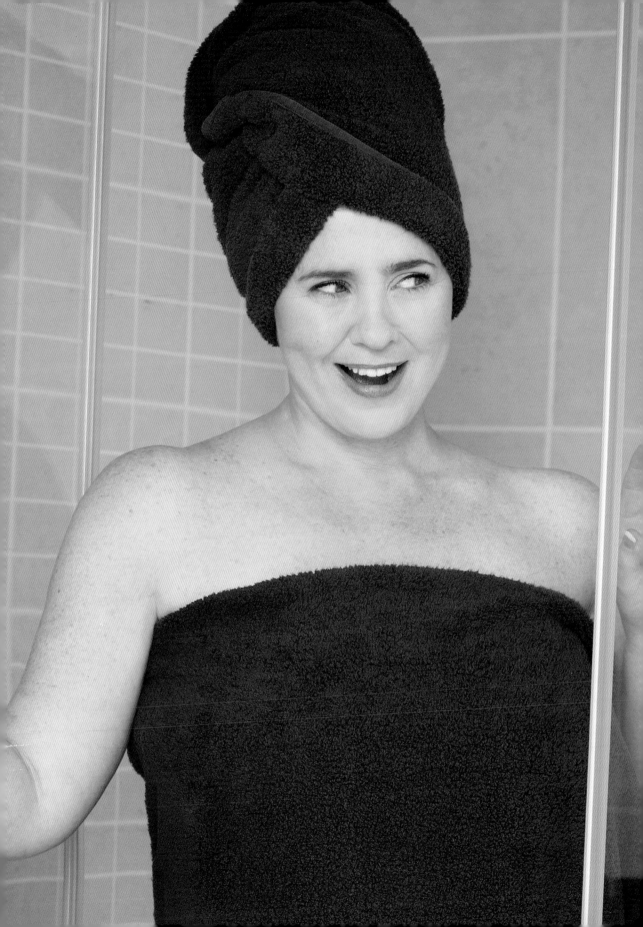

Save £435 a Year!

Yes, unbelievably that's what it could cost you to keep your hair in great shape colour-wise at a salon. Colouring your hair at home is not difficult; just remember these tips:

➤ *Choose your colour well and make sure you spend some time examining the colour charts on the packaging.*

➤ *Always do the allergy and strand tests, as instructed by the manufacturer. I know it seems a bore and you want to colour your hair **now**, but if you haven't used the brand or shade before you need to know how your hair and skin will react.*

➤ *Smear Vaseline along your hairline to prevent the dye from running and staining your skin. Keep a cotton-wool ball handy to mop up smudges as you go along as hair colour can be very difficult to remove.*

➤ *Wear the plastic gloves provided, use an old towel and follow the instructions to the letter.*

➤ *If you want to cover grey hair, colour this area first; it will need longer to take.*

➤ *Remember that permed hair is more porous and will soak up the colour faster, so wait a couple of weeks after perming before colouring your hair. You will also achieve better results on well-conditioned hair, so it might be wise to have a trim beforehand, too.*

THE PERFECT BLOW-DRY

THERE'S NOTHING QUITE LIKE HAVING YOUR HAIR BLOW-DRIED BY A PROFESSIONAL. YEARS OF PRACTICE, THE RIGHT TOOLS AND NOT HAVING TO WORK WITH THEIR HANDS BEHIND THEIR HEAD MEAN THEY CAN ACHIEVE RESULTS YOU CAN ONLY DREAM OF.

But it's not impossible to give yourself the near-professional treatment. When I'm working I'm lucky to have the experts on hand, although more often than not it's heated rollers and cans of hairspray that create the finished look. At home, though, I can be out of the shower, with hair dried and shiny in fifteen minutes.

HERE'S HOW I DO IT:

1 I make sure I condition my hair each time I wash it. Once out of the shower I blot the excess water from my hair without rubbing too hard.

2 I squeeze a small amount of hair serum onto my palm and work it through my hair, starting at the ends.

3 Then I use a wide-toothed comb to spread the serum evenly through my hair and get rid of any tangles.

4 Next I use my hairdryer on a medium setting to remove 80 per cent of the moisture. I always make sure the nozzle is on my dryer.

5 I clip my hair onto the top of my head, leaving the underneath layers to be dried first. I make sure I'm sitting comfortably so that when I raise my arms they don't ache too quickly.

6 I direct the dryer down the shafts of my hair and use a wide, flat paddle brush with natural bristles to create a smooth style. If I want to bend my hair under or out, or give it volume, I use a round brush.

7 Gradually unclipping my damp hair, I work from the back of my head to the front, drying small sections at a time.

8 I always finish with the hair around my face – I find that the tricky bit – and I make sure my hair is completely dry before turning off the heat.

9 A quick blast on the cold-air button is good for 'setting' the style, particularly if I'm going for a straight, shiny look.

Variations on this include my 'upside-down' look, when I bend over at the waist and dry my hair from the roots. It's great when you want extra volume. I also try to let my hair dry naturally as often as possible, just to give my poor hair an occasional rest!

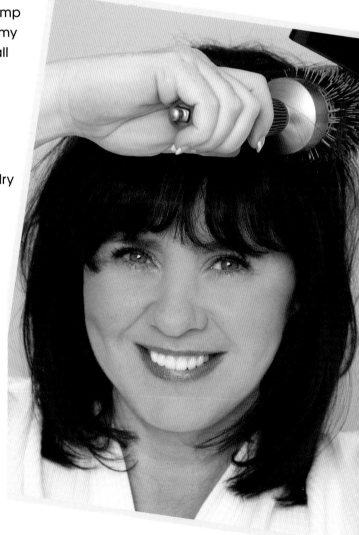

IT'S A CRUEL, CRUEL WORLD!

AND TALKING OF GIVING YOUR HAIR A REST, IT'S ESPECIALLY IMPORTANT TO GO FOR THE NATURAL LOOK ONCE IN A WHILE IF YOU REGULARLY INFLICT EXTRA HEAT ON YOUR TRESSES, IN THE FORM OF STRAIGHTENING IRONS, HEATED ROLLERS OR CURLING TONGS.

All these appliances are brilliant for creating smooth, shiny styles or wild, wild curls, but they do take their toll on your locks. If you can afford them, opt for ceramic straightening irons, as these will be kinder to your hair. And never straighten without drying first. Finally, don't forget to use a heat protection spray or cream – your hair will thank you for it.

AS IF BY MAGIC!

THE EAGLE-EYED AMONG YOU MAY HAVE NOTICED THAT MY HAIR SOMETIMES GROWS SUPER QUICKLY. NO, I HAVEN'T DISCOVERED A

WONDER GROWTH SERUM; THE ANSWER LIES IN HAIR EXTENSIONS. I DON'T MIND ADMITTING THAT I LIKE AN EXTENSION OR TWO, JUST TO GIVE MY OWN HAIR A LITTLE EXTRA VOLUME OR LENGTH WHEN I FANCY IT.

During The Nolans' tour I used a half-wig – the fringe was all my own but I borrowed the rest of my long, straight style. It gets so hot on stage that before long you're really sweaty, and that's when my hair starts misbehaving and sticking to my head. Off-stage, though, I just use a couple of clip-on extensions.

These extensions have become really popular lately – and you don't need to spend a fortune having your hairdresser put them in at the salon. Clip-on hair pieces are much more affordable and don't damage your real hair because it's not necessary to use heat or glue to apply them; they simply clip invisibly onto your own locks. It could be you fancy having longer hair for a special occasion, or you might have very fine hair and want some added fullness – either way, clip-on extensions could be the answer. To find out more, ask your hairdresser for advice or take a look in your nearest good department store. Go on, be brave!

INSTANT GLAMOUR

HAIRBANDS ARE NOT JUST FOR LITTLE GIRLS AND POSH PEOPLE, YOU KNOW.

These days you'll find department-store counters full of sparkly clips, glittery slides, Grecian bands, flowers, bows and butterflies that look great on women of any age. For a really special occasion there are beautiful tiaras and fascinators (feathers, netting or sparkly bows on a stiff headband), or you could go for a ponytail hairpiece. The possibilities are endless.

HELP YOURSELF FOR FREE

YOU COULD GET LOST AMONG THE THOUSANDS OF HAIR PRODUCTS AVAILABLE IN THE SHOPS. THERE ARE SO MANY DIFFERENT BRANDS, ALL DOING DIFFERENT JOBS, AND ALL WITH A HEFTY PRICE TAG ATTACHED. I ALWAYS BUY A MID-PRICED, GENTLE SHAMPOO AND CONDITIONER AND OCCASIONALLY I'LL FORK OUT FOR A HAIR COLOUR. THE REST OF MY HAIR TREATMENTS, HOWEVER, I CAN FIND IN MY OWN KITCHEN CUPBOARDS.

Banana and Honey Shine

Mash together a banana with one tablespoon of clear, runny honey. Apply over wet hair, cover with a warm towel and leave for an hour. Shampoo and rinse well. Leaves your hair looking beautifully glossy.

No More Frizz

Shampoo, rinse and towel-dry your hair. Mash half an avocado with a tablespoon of mayonnaise, apply from root to tip and leave for ten minutes. Rinse well. This will deeply moisturise your hair and calm frizz by smoothing the hair shaft.

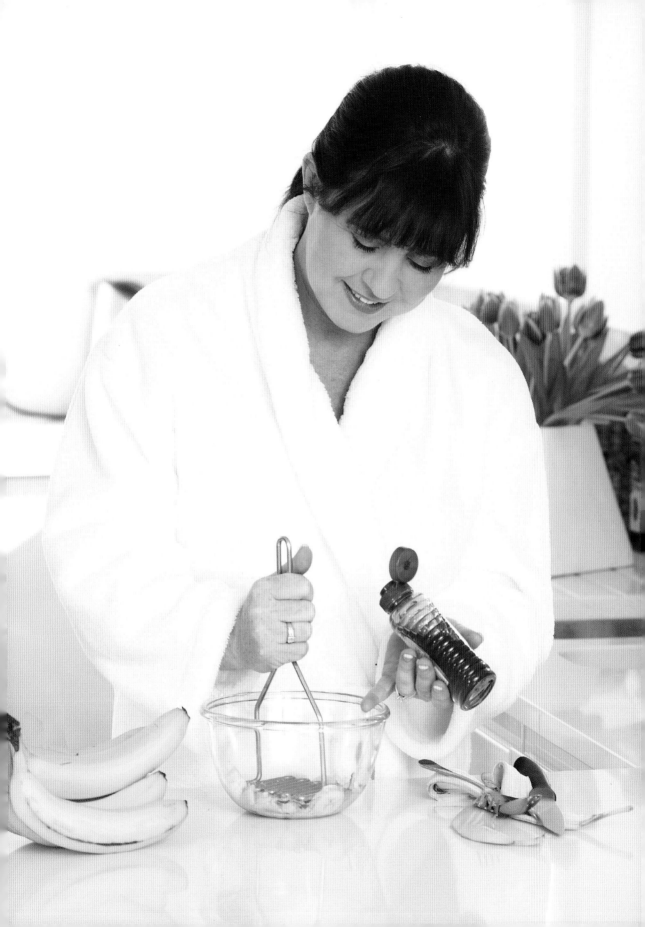

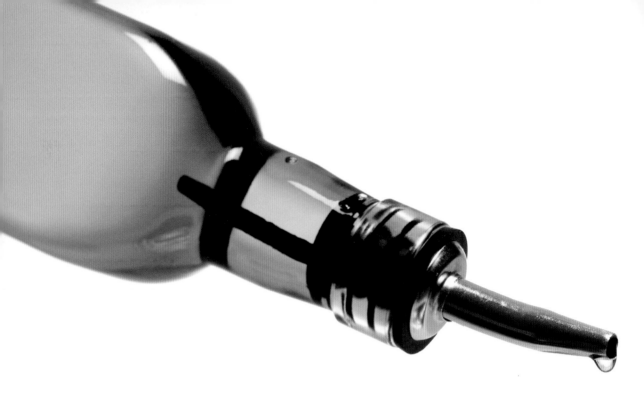

Olive Oil and Egg Conditioning Mask

Mix four tablespoons of olive oil with a beaten egg. Apply to wet hair and cover with a warm towel. Leave on the hair for up to an hour, then shampoo and rinse well. Does wonders for dry hair.

Mayonnaise Conditioner

After shampooing, massage ordinary mayonnaise into your hair. Leave it on for fifteen minutes, then lightly shampoo again and rinse well. Your hair will feel really soft after this treatment.

Tropical Treat

Mash an avocado with a little coconut milk for a smooth, runny consistency. Apply to your hair and leave on for fifteen minutes, then shampoo as normal. Leaves your hair in wonderful condition.

Honey Conditioner

Mix two parts clear, runny honey to one part olive oil and apply to wet hair. Comb through with a wide-toothed comb. Cover your head with a warm towel and leave for thirty minutes. Shampoo and rinse well. Adds shine to dry or dull hair.

'BEER IS EXCELLENT FOR KEEPING YOUR HAIR STRONG AND SHINY – AND DON'T WORRY, YOU WON'T SMELL LIKE A BREWERY AFTERWARDS'

● *Rosemary for Brunettes*

For shiny dark hair, try this herby rinse. Pour boiling water over fresh rosemary, let it brew for ten minutes, then cool the liquid by adding some cold water. Use as a rinse after shampooing and conditioning, letting it sit on the hair for five minutes before giving your hair a final rinse.

● *Camomile for Blondes*

If you are blonde, get the same shiny effect by brewing up some camomile tea. Make sure you cool the liquid down before using it, then rinse.

● *Vinegar Rinse*

Wash and condition your hair as usual, then mix one part cider or wine vinegar to four parts water and use as a final rinse. Leaves you with super shiny locks.

● *Egg Conditioner*

Add one teaspoon of baby oil to a beaten egg yolk, then beat again and add sixteen tablespoons of water. Shampoo as normal, then massage the egg conditioner into the scalp for a few minutes and rinse well.

● *Mine's a Pint*

Beer is excellent for keeping your hair strong and shiny – and don't worry, you won't smell like a brewery afterwards. Just massage any dark beer – bitter or stout – into clean, wet, shampooed hair. Cover your head with a warm towel and leave for ten minutes, then condition as normal. Cheers!

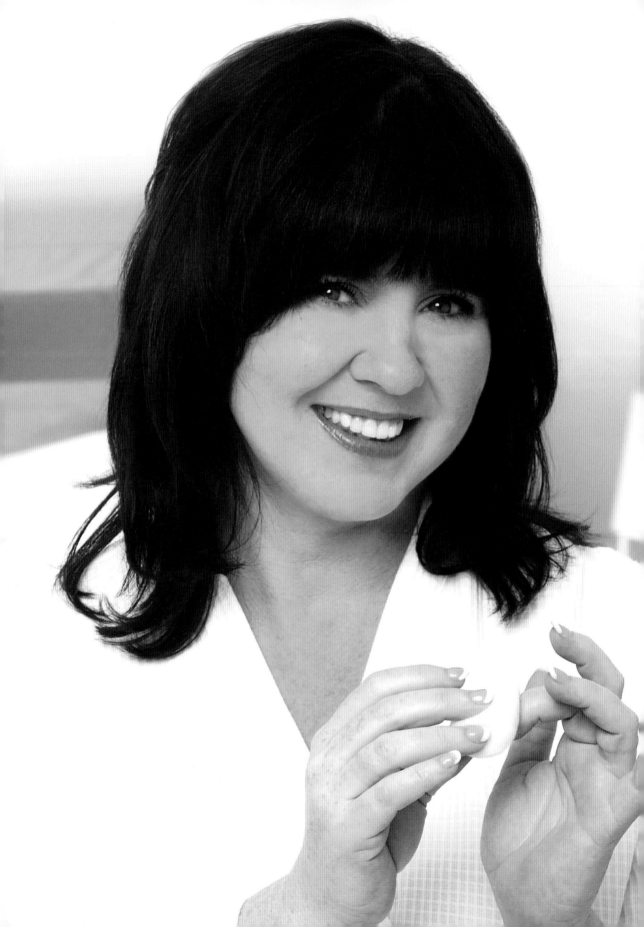

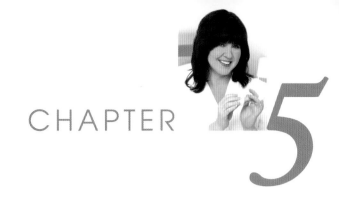

CHAPTER 5

*Touch me in
the morning...*

YOUR HANDS
AND FEET

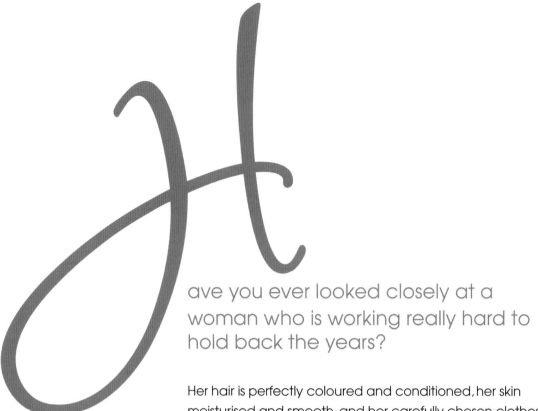

Have you ever looked closely at a woman who is working really hard to hold back the years?

Her hair is perfectly coloured and conditioned, her skin moisturised and smooth, and her carefully chosen clothes wouldn't look out of place on a woman in her thirties. Everything about her tells you she's yet to tackle middle age – until you look down and see the hands of a seventy-year-old. Yes, neglect your hands and you may as well wear a badge with your age on it.

Our hands – and, in the summer, our feet – have been exposed to all weathers. They've washed dishes, cleaned toilets, changed babies' nappies and fetched and carried for as long as we've been around. Is it any wonder, then, that they are usually the first bit of our body to show their age or perhaps look even older than we are?

Our hands are furthest away from our central circulatory system and the skin on them is thin, delicate and often dry. Meanwhile our feet suffer years of abuse from high heels, neglect and wear and tear. Don't be surprised, then, if you look down one day and see a pair of specimens straight out of *Lord of the Rings*!

> '**NEGLECT YOUR HANDS AND YOU MAY AS WELL WEAR A BADGE WITH YOUR AGE ON IT**'

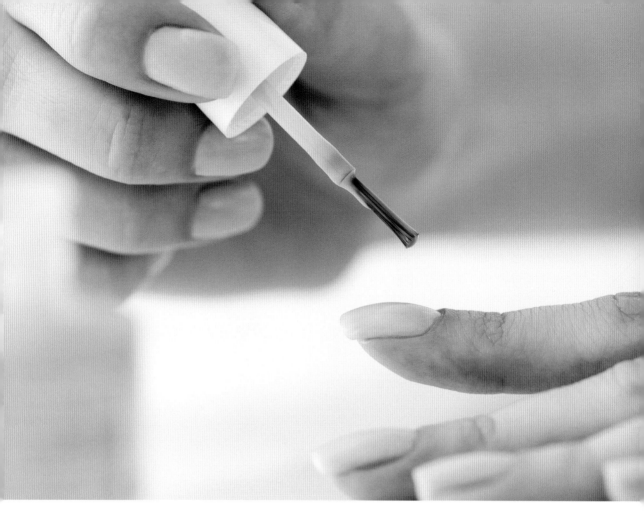

I once worked out that I could quite easily spend fourteen hours a week with my hands in the sink, yet I could never find the time to have a manicure. And as for my feet, well, until I lost weight I couldn't even see them, and I'm afraid it was a case of out of sight, out of mind. The word pedicure honestly never entered my head until recently.

Once I began to look after the rest of my body, however, I realised I wanted to take care of every bit of me. Not just my face and hair, but those bits that were, quite literally, stuck out on a limb. I realised that I didn't necessarily need to spend money on professional manicures and pedicures – I could pamper my own hands and feet quickly, cheaply and without fuss.

And the result? Manicures and pretty nails give me pleasure, while pedicures and healthy feet give me energy. And when the summer begins I don't have to cover up in case someone mistakes me for a hobbit!

HANDS

I DON'T THINK ANYONE REALLY LOVES THEIR OWN HANDS, DO THEY? WHEN I LOOK AT MINE I WISH THEY WERE SLENDER, WITH LONG, ELEGANT FINGERS.

My hands have always been the same shape, even after I lost 5 stone. Mind you, if I had to choose I'd lose fat off my bum anytime. Since I began taking better care of my hands I have definitely noticed my skin tone improving. I used to suffer from dry, flaky skin, but now that my hands are well moisturised, the wrinkles that went with the dry skin have vanished.

As for my nails, I'm ashamed to say I've treated them appallingly. I have good, strong hair – thanks again, Mum – and, as we have already said, hair and nails are made of the same material, so my nails should have been strong and healthy if I'd given them the chance. Instead I've bitten them to the quick since I was a child, and now I've started hiding them away under gel nail extensions. Luckily false nails are so amazingly realistic that nobody spots my guilty secret.

When I think of how often my hands are on show – holding a microphone on the TV in front of thousands or stroking Ciara's hair as she falls asleep – I'm very glad they no longer let me down. False nails aren't for everybody, though, and later on in this chapter I'll give you some tips on how to encourage your own nails to grow longer and stronger.

A Soft Touch

HERE'S A VERY SIMPLE TEST THAT WILL TELL YOU IF YOUR HANDS ARE DEHYDRATED:

Gently pinch the skin on the back of your hand and see how long it takes to fall back into place. If it's longer than a second, then your skin needs moisture. If you want to take this test a little further, pinch for five seconds, then count how long it takes for the skin to return to its original place.

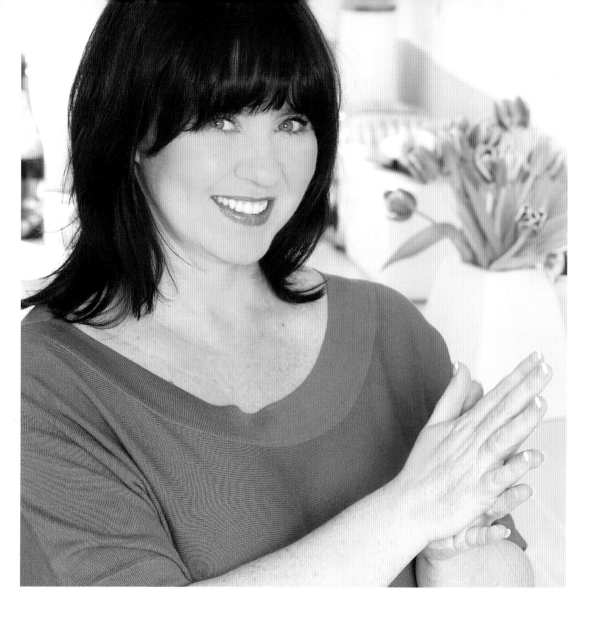

The experts say you can tell your skin's age by the number of seconds this takes. Try it and see if your skin is **YOUNGER, OLDER** or **IN LINE** with your biological age.

TIME (IN SECONDS)

- *1–2 (under 30 years old)*
- *3–4 (30–44 years old)*
- *5–9 (45–50 years old)*
- *10–15 (60 years old)*
- *16 or more (70 years old)*

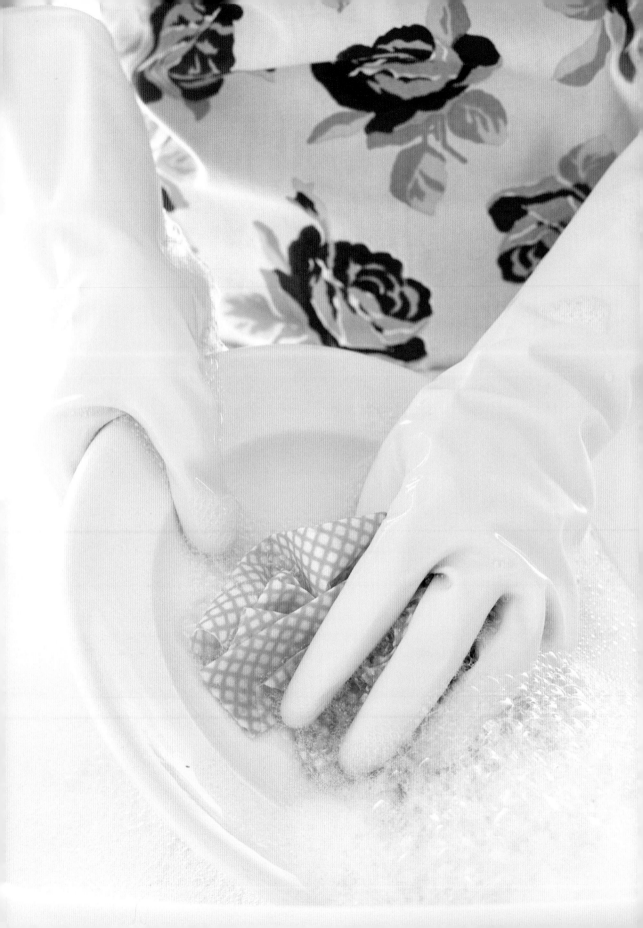

Don't worry if you're still waiting for your skin to lie flat! The good news is that with some TLC your hands can become beautiful once more.

FOLLOW THESE SIMPLE RULES AND YOU'LL SOON SEE SMOOTHER SKIN EMERGING:

1 It's the old SPF nag again. Always use a hand cream with a protection factor of at least 15, especially in the summer, or use sunscreen on top of your usual moisturiser. The sun's harmful rays will damage the delicate skin on your hands and leave them dry and wrinkled, while protecting the skin on your hands from sun damage will prevent unsightly age spots in the future.

2 In the winter, keep your hands warm with gloves. Extreme cold is just as harmful as extreme high temperatures.

3 Don't forget your Marigolds. Always use protective gloves when doing household jobs – it's obvious the damage that can be done by harsh chemicals, but even long sessions in water can be harmful.

4 Keep some hand cream next to each sink in your house and use it every time you dry your hands. You can't over-moisturise the skin on your hands, so get used to doing it several times a day and your hands will thank you for it. My sister Maureen is never without hand cream and puts it on regularly during the day, and she has the softest skin I've ever felt; it's like a baby's.

5 If your hands are very dry, try fixing them in your sleep. Just before you put your head on the pillow apply some rich hand cream and pull on some light cotton gloves – ignoring the look of alarm on your partner's face! By morning they will be thoroughly moisturised.

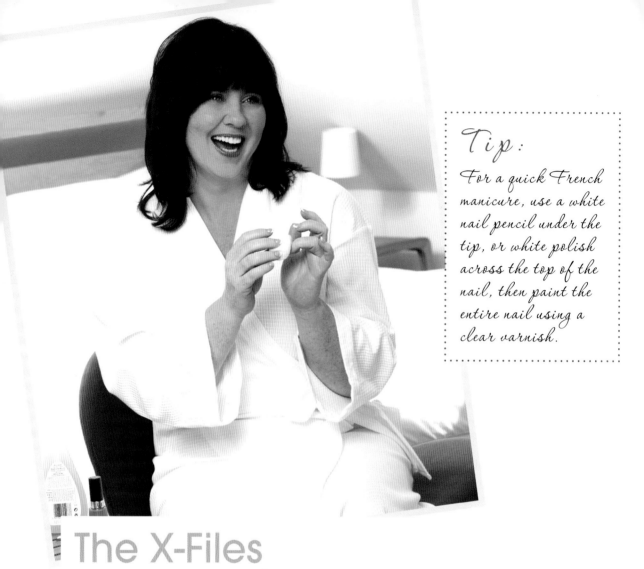

Tip:

For a quick French manicure, use a white nail pencil under the tip, or white polish across the top of the nail, then paint the entire nail using a clear varnish.

The X-Files

Occasionally, if I'm in need of some pampering, I treat myself to a professional manicure to hide my horribly bitten nails. It's quite easy to find a salon on the high street, and it's not that expensive to pop in for a little pampering. But the problem is that once you're short of time or cash, spending either on simply filing your nails feels a bit daft. And the next thing you know you're back to raggedy nails, leathery cuticles and hands like a bricklayer's.

These days I give myself a weekly manicure that never takes more than thirty minutes. I find it quite relaxing and it can be done while slumped on the sofa watching *Coronation Street*. It's also a lovely thing to do for someone else, too, and as I'm lucky enough to have a daughter, Ciara and I often spend a girly night together filing our nails and choosing nail-polish colours.

YOU WILL NEED: *nail polish remover, cotton wool, a bowl of warm soapy water, an orange stick, a nail file and nail polish. (It will take a little more time and money, but I really do think it's worth also using a nail base coat and a top coat.)*

The Perfect, Easy Manicure

- First, file your nails into shape, choosing a rounded or a squared shape – I think a square edge looks a bit more modern. Whatever the shape, file from one outside edge to the centre and then from the other edge back to the centre. Don't file in both directions as this will damage the nail.

- Remove all traces of your old nail polish using nail varnish remover on a ball of cotton wool.

- Soak your hands in the soapy water for at least five minutes. Make sure the water isn't too hot – you want it just warm enough to soften the cuticles. Dry well.

- Wrap a small amount of cotton wool around the tip of the orange stick and gently push back your cuticles. This makes the nail look longer, as well as making it easier to apply the polish. Take care not to break the cuticle and never cut it.

- Lie your hand flat and brush on a layer of base coat. This will stop the coloured polish from staining your nails and make it easier to apply the varnish. Allow to dry for a few minutes.

- Apply the colour. Brush a single stroke down the middle of the nail, then one on either side. Don't worry if you haven't gone right to the outside edge – a small gap will make your nail look longer. Paint down to the cuticle but don't get polish on the skin. If you make a mistake, keep an orange stick tipped with some cotton wool soaked in varnish remover to hand. Allow your nails to dry and then, if you have time, apply a second coat. Make sure the varnish is dry – about three minutes should do it – before moving on to the final stage. Alternatively, use a clear polish and avoid colour clashes with your clothes.

- Finish off with a top coat. This will seal the polish and also stop the colour from chipping.

Naughty Nibbles

Are you a nail-biter like me? I don't know what makes us do it. Is it nerves? Boredom? Hunger?! Bitten nails look awful and I always try to wear false gel extensions if I'm going out. I remember feeling terrible once at a posh do because, although I was wearing a beautiful gown and my hair and make-up were perfect, I hadn't had time to get my nails done. I was so embarrassed.

When I was a kid my mum tried every trick in the book to get me to stop nibbling my nails. She put a sticking plaster around every fingertip, but I just pulled them off; even that vile-tasting liquid didn't deter me. After all these years I'm still trying to kick the habit.

PERHAPS YOU'LL HAVE BETTER LUCK WITH THESE REMEDIES:

- Next time you find yourself biting your nails, make a note of what you are doing and when. It could be that you only nibble when you're hungry, or feeling stressed. Identify the cause and try to avoid these situations.

- Use a foul-tasting solution on your nails – the bitterness should deter you from putting your fingers in your mouth.

- Embark on a nail campaign. Choose one fingernail and let it grow, then another, then another and so on. Once you see how nice your nails can look it will encourage you to grow the others.

- Keep your nails painted – it's definitely not as nice chomping away on nails covered in varnish.

- Have a nail file handy. Sometimes we nibble just to even out a rough or broken nail, but if you keep a file in your handbag, you can repair damaged nails instead of destroying them.

- Set a goal. A wedding is a great incentive, even if you are only a guest. Alternatively, aim to grow your nails in time for a holiday or a big social event.

- If you really can't kick the habit, consider getting a set of false nails, either a

DIY shop-bought pack or a set of acrylic or gel nails at your local nail salon. Falsies are an extreme solution as they can often do more harm to your real nails than good, but they taste revolting, so they may just break your nail-biting cycle.

Long and Strong

Even if we don't bite our nails, some of us find it difficult to grow them. Often nails are too soft or easily damaged. You can buy nail-strengthening kits, but they're expensive.

WHY NOT TRY THESE OPTIONS FIRST:

● Did you know that stimulating the circulation around your fingernail encourages growth? That's why the fingernails on your writing hand grow faster than the nails on your other hand. Massage the base of your nails with oil – olive oil will do – to stimulate your circulation as often as you can.

● Look at your diet. As with your hair and your skin, a poor diet can have a dramatic effect on the health and appearance of your nails. Dry, brittle fingernails could be lacking vitamin A, which can be found in liver and oily fish; cracked nails could be caused by dehydration – are you drinking enough water? – ridges on your nails may be due to lack of iron, which you get from red meat and dark green vegetables, and weak nails could be caused by a lack of calcium in your diet, which you can boost by having more milk and cheese. A good supply of protein – found in meat, nuts, beans and eggs – will also improve the health of your nails.

● Change your shampoo. If you're using a shampoo designed to strip oil from greasy hair, it could be drying out your fingernails, too. Experiment with different products and see if your nails improve.

● Go naked! Give your nails a rest for a few days a month – no varnish, no strengtheners, no harsh removers. Simply file and moisturise as usual and let your nails breathe.

FEET

YOU'VE GOT TO FEEL SORRY FOR FEET. THEY'RE OFTEN COMPLETELY NEGLECTED, GET SHOVED INTO RIDICULOUS SHOES AND CARRY US AROUND FROM MORNING TILL NIGHT.

And who loves them? Show me a man or woman with a fetish for feet and I'll show you someone who's a bit, well, odd. I made a discovery recently, though. You don't have to like anyone else's feet – although babies' toes are delicious, aren't they? – but if you begin to love yours a little more, they will repay you in spades. Take some time to look after your tootsies and they will give you more energy, extra confidence and the quiet satisfaction that you have the prettiest feet in the room. The alternative is just too grim: aching, tired, painful, unattractive and unloved feet are a curse.

HERE'S HOW TO AVOID THEM:

- KEEP THEM CLEAN. You need to wash your feet thoroughly every day. Don't forget to clean between each toe, then dry them well so there are no warm, moist areas where harmful bacteria can hide.

- REMOVE HARD SKIN. Whether you use a pumice stone, a foot file or exfoliating cream, don't let hard skin build up as this will lead to cracked, painful and unattractive heels.

- DON'T NEGLECT YOUR NAILS. A regular pedicure at home will ensure your nails are kept in shape and you'll avoid ingrowing toenails and infections.

- MOISTURISE! Keep the skin on your feet silky smooth. The sole of your foot is very thick so you'll need a rich, intensive moisturiser that can soak into this area.

- DON'T DO A POSH. Victoria Beckham has everything in the world that she wants, but she also has painful-looking bunions, probably caused by wearing impossibly high shoes every day of her life. High heels look sexy, but if you alternate them with more sensible shoes, you'll save yourself a lot of discomfort.

- Let your feet breathe. Kick off your shoes and go barefoot whenever possible.

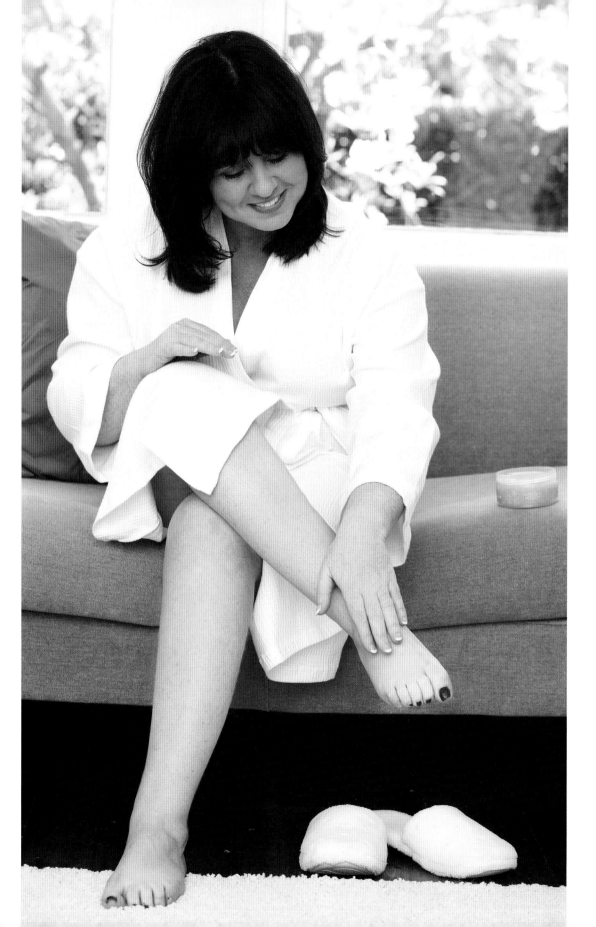

Six Steps to Heaven

It took me years to be brave enough to let someone else touch my feet, but once I'd experienced my first pedicure there was no going back – I left that salon feeling as if I was walking on air. Not many of us have the time or money to spend lolling around in spas having our feet massaged, but there's no reason why you can't do it yourself at home. Or better still, teach your partner how to give you the perfect pedicure – it really is blissful.

YOU WILL NEED: *a bowl of warm soapy water, a clean fluffy towel, nail clippers, a nail file, an orange stick, a cotton-wool bud, a pumice stone or foot file, and moisturiser.*

The Perfect, Easy Pedicure

- First, soak your feet in warm soapy water for between five and ten minutes.

- Take the pumice stone or foot file and gently rub at the areas of thicker, hard skin. Never be tempted to cut this away instead, as it will just be replaced by even tougher skin.

- Use the nail clippers to trim your toenails, cutting straight across to avoid ingrowing nails. You can then use the nail file to smooth any rough edges.

- Wrap a small amount of cotton wool around the tip of the orange stick and gently push back the cuticles of your toenails. Use the stick to clean under your nails.

- Now comes the blissful bit. Smooth moisturiser all over your foot and massage for at least five minutes. Try not to rush this part of the pedicure.

- If you like polish on your toenails, wipe away any excess moisturiser and apply clear or coloured varnish, following the same steps as for the manicure. A topcoat isn't really necessary as you're not likely to chip the colour, but it will make your toenails shiny.

Tip: Store your nail varnish in the fridge. It will last longer and you'll be able to apply it more smoothly.

Kick Those Problems

I can't be happy if my feet are giving me trouble. Here's a quick look at some of the most common problems and how to solve them:

● *Cracked Heels*

You can prevent this with regular pumice-stone sessions followed by lots of moisturising foot cream. If you've already got cracked heels, you may need to buy a foot balm from the chemist. There are plenty out there; the trick is making sure you use the treatment daily until the hard skin is gone.

● *Bunions*

Painful and unsightly, bunions are a deformity of the big toe joint and are usually hereditary, although wearing tight shoes and high heels will make the problem worse. The only solution is surgery, so ask your GP for advice.

● *Yellow Toenails*

This is staining caused by using dark polish on your nails. Try using a base coat first, switching to paler shades or letting your nails go naked for a while.

● *Smelly Feet*

Never wear shoes or trainers that are still damp with sweat; keep your feet clean and always wear fresh socks or tights. If your feet are really sweaty, try wiping them clean with cotton wool dipped in surgical spirit. You should also check for fungal infections between your toes and on the soles of your feet.

● *Athlete's Foot*

If you have itchy, inflamed skin, you may have this fungal infection. Ask your chemist for advice.

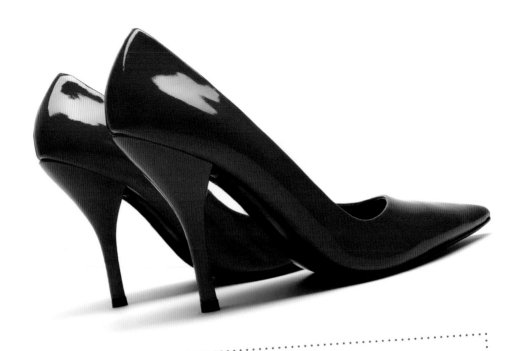

Oh, My Aching Feet!

There's nothing like a pair of sexy high heels to complete an evening outfit – a posh dress doesn't really look right without them – but once I get that burning sensation in the ball of my foot I have to ditch the stilettos. I'm always the first to sit down and take my shoes off under the table – and nine times out of ten I end up losing one of them!

I've noticed this pain getting worse as I've got older, and that's because as the body matures you naturally lose fat on the ball of your foot. Typical isn't it, the one place you need a bit of padding and it automatically slims down as you age!

Celebrity stylists recommend using gel pads as they replace the fat padding you lose under your feet. They also advise shopping carefully for shoes and making sure you try before you buy – a pair of shoes that make your feet slide forward will cripple you on a big night out.

My advice, though, is to always take a second pair of shoes out with you. On many nights I've kissed the flip-flops I've hidden in my handbag!

'ON MANY NIGHTS I'VE KISSED THE FLIP-FLOPS I'VE HIDDEN IN MY HANDBAG!'

Treat Your Toes

Now your feet are so pretty you can begin to enjoy them! If you've never had a foot massage it's time to discover what you've been missing. Either give yourself a massage or find a volunteer to do it for you. You'll need a comfortable chair, a warm room and some peace and quiet; candles and soft music won't hurt either.

HERE'S HOW I DO IT:

- Smooth oil onto your feet – it doesn't have to be expensive massage oil; baby or olive oil will do. Start at your toes and apply up to your ankle.

- With the tips of your fingers, use long, gentle strokes to massage the top, the sides and the sole of your foot.

- Push your thumb under your toes, then slide your fingers between each one and gently move each toe in a circle.

- Now firmly run your thumb along your inner arch, from the heel to the big toe. Repeat on the outside edge from the heel to the little toe.

- Hold your Achilles tendon – the band of tissue that goes from your calf muscle to your heel – between thumb and forefinger and stroke downwards.

- Use your thumb to make firm circles on the ball of your foot, the arch and your heel.

- Stretch each toe, pulling gently with your thumb and forefinger. Now go back and repeat, this time gliding your fingers off the end of the toes. Bliss!

HELP YOURSELF FOR FREE

YOU DON'T HAVE TO SPEND A FORTUNE ON YOUR HANDS AND FEET; JUST GIVE THEM A LITTLE TENDER LOVING CARE USING INGREDIENTS YOU'LL ALREADY HAVE IN THE HOUSE. WHY NOT TRY THESE CLEVER EXERCISES TO KEEP YOUR FINGERS FLEXIBLE AND YOUR FEET AS LIGHT AS A FEATHER:

● *Hand Manoeuvres*

Try these hand exercises to release tension and keep your fingers strong and mobile:

➧ *Find a small rubber ball – keep it next to the chair you sit in to watch telly, perhaps – and squeeze it in both hands whenever you remember.*

➧ *Lay your hand on a flat surface, spread your fingers, then raise your wrist as far as possible while leaving your fingers flat on the surface.*

➧ *Try playing 'air piano', holding your hands in the air and using your fingers to play imaginary notes.*

➧ *Practise writing with the hand you don't normally use.*

● *Fancy Footwork*

These exercises will keep your feet strong and take away the stresses of the day. Do them as often as you can and you will soon feel the difference.

➡ Roll a golf ball under your bare foot for two minutes each side, making firm circular movements from the ball of the foot to the arch and then to the heel.

➡ Point your toes and raise your leg, then write the letters of the alphabet in the air.

➡ Use your toes to pick up small objects – a pencil, for example – and place them in a container.

➡ Put a rubber band round both big toes and pull your feet apart. Hold for five seconds, then relax.

Cuticle Softener

Mix one teaspoon of runny honey with two teaspoons of lemon juice and half a cup of warm water. Soak your fingers in the liquid for up to fifteen minutes and gently dry before manicuring. You should now find it much easier to push back your cuticles.

Nail Strengthener

Gelatin is great for weak nails; in fact I've heard stories of people eating a cube of jelly a day to keep their nails in good shape. Mix a packet of powdered gelatin with a little hot water, keep the mixture thick, then dunk your fingertips in it. Soak for at least fifteen minutes, then rinse and dry for super-strength nails.

Oaty Hand Scrub

Soak two tablespoons of porridge oats in two fluid ounces of warm water and leave for five minutes while the oats soften. Add one and a half teaspoons of lemon juice and half a teaspoon of olive oil and mix well. Massage the oats into your hands for at least two minutes, then rinse with warm water. Dry well and finish with a moisturiser. Leaves skin feeling soft and supple.

Hand Softener

Put a large knob of soft butter and a spoonful of brown sugar into the palms of your hands, then rub together for ten minutes. Rinse with warm water, dry and moisturise. Will leave your hands feeling really smooth.

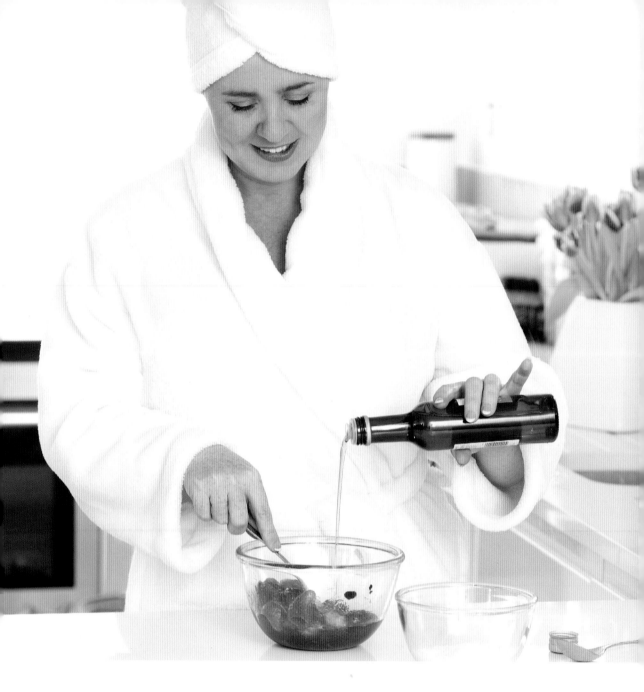

● *Hand and Foot Strawberry Treat*

This recipe is good for the skin on your hands and feet. It's a bit of a luxury to use strawberries, but next time you have some that are past their best, try this. Mix ten strawberries with two tablespoons of olive oil and a teaspoon of coarse sea salt. Massage into your hands and feet, rinse with warm water, dry and moisturise. It will leave your skin feeling and smelling wonderful.

Hand Mask

Peel a banana and place it and half of the skin in a food processor, along with a tablespoon of runny honey. Blend and smooth the paste onto your hands, then leave until it's dry. Wash off with warm water, dry and moisturise. This really nourishes dry skin, leaving it feeling soft and silky.

Sugary Hand Rub

Combine three spoonfuls of sugar with vegetable or olive oil and massage firmly into your hands and fingers, using the thumb and forefinger of the opposite hand. Rub in for around five minutes before rinsing with warm water and moisturising.

Milky Foot Soaker

Boil half a litre of milk with 1.5 litres of water, then turn the heat off and add 120ml of sugar and two tablespoons of body lotion. Mix well and pour into a washing-up bowl. When the liquid is cool enough, use as a foot bath. Soak your feet for fifteen minutes then rinse, dry and moisturise. It's the perfect pick-me-up for tired feet.

Foot Scrub

Soak your feet for five minutes in warm water, then massage using a thick paste of coarse sea salt and olive oil. The oil will make your toenails shine, while the sea salt will act as an exfoliator, leaving your feet feeling lovely and soft. Rinse, then moisturise.

Coffee Foot Scrub

Mix four tablespoons of used coffee grounds with three tablespoons of porridge oats, three tablespoons of coarse sea salt and three tablespoons of olive oil. Use the mixture to scrub your feet, then rinse with warm water, dry and moisturise. This is great for dry and cracked heels, but will leave any foot feeling fantastic.

Sandy Toes

Have you ever noticed how good your feet feel after you've been on holiday? It's because the sand on the beach gently exfoliates any dry skin. Next time you're near a beach take a small container of sand back home with you and use it to treat your feet all year long. Just mix together equal measures of sand and baby oil and massage into your feet, concentrating on any dry areas. Rinse and moisturise.

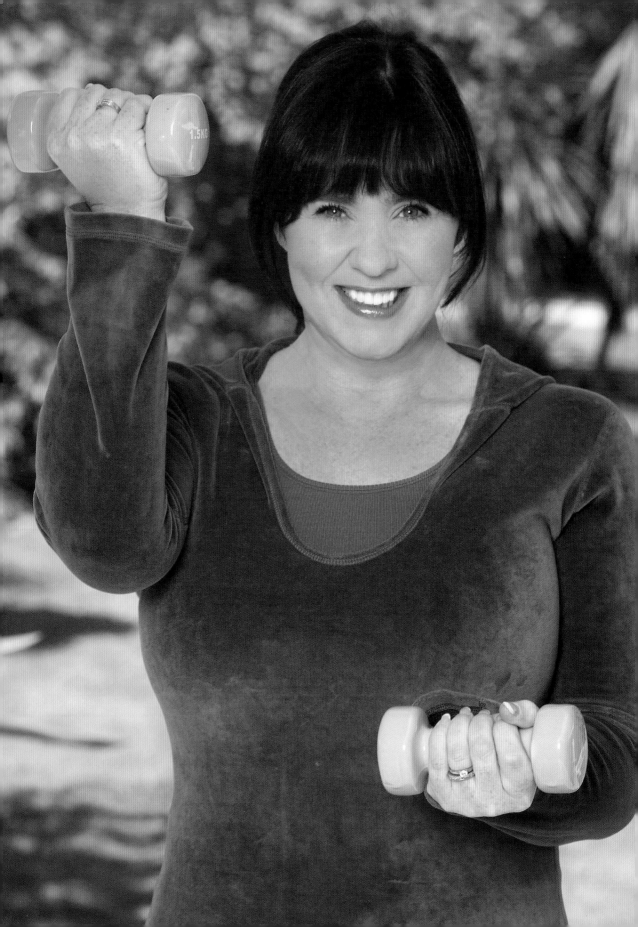

CHAPTER 6

Let's get physical....

EXERCISE
AND DIET

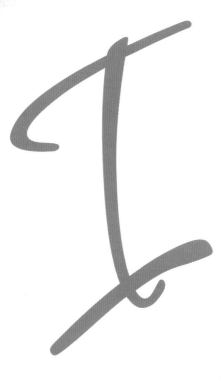**I** could have kissed the *Dancing on Ice* physio who told me not to run any more because it was bad for my dodgy knee.

It was as good as being told that I'd given birth to a healthy, bouncing baby. But even as I was hanging up my running shoes, I knew that I would have to replace the dreaded jog with some other form of exercise or the pounds would start piling on again.

As I've already mentioned, I've lost weight several times in my life, but until recently I hadn't found a way to keep it off. I suppose the answer was always right there in front of me, I was just too fed up and unhappy to see it. Even the smallest amount of exercise – because that, I'm afraid, ladies, is the only answer – can seem like a massive mountain to climb when you're in a rut and lacking confidence.

But before you raise your eyes and turn to the next chapter…

'IT'S POSSIBLE FOR EXERCISE TO BE FUN, PAINLESS AND EXHILARATING'

STOP!

I'll let you into a secret…it doesn't have to be torture. Honestly. It is possible to build regular exercise into your daily routine, and it is possible for that exercise to be fun, painless and exhilarating.

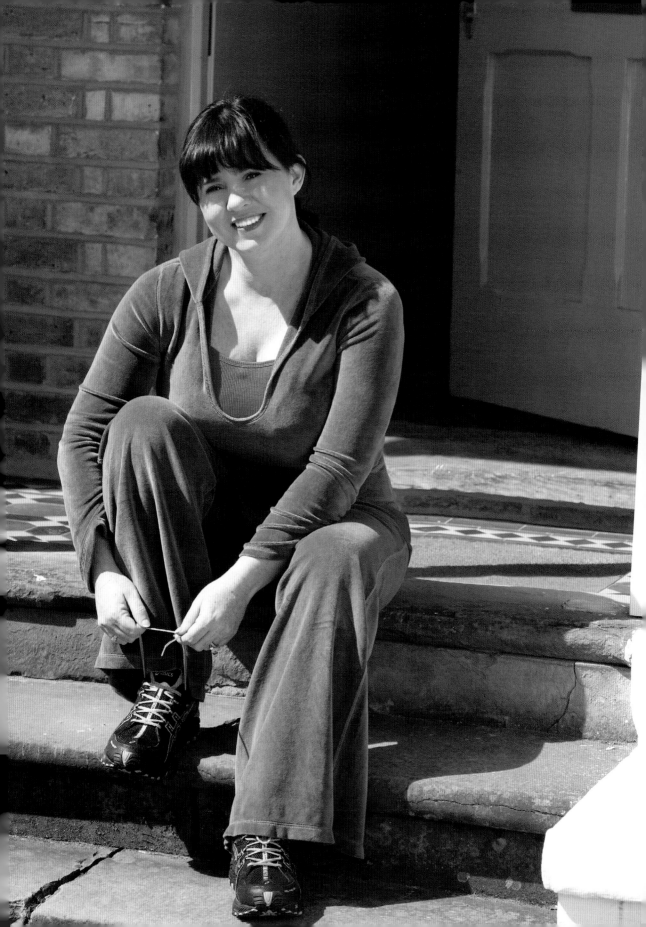

You don't have to pound the streets jogging – with my weak knee and 36FF boobs, I was either going to end up on crutches or with two black eyes. And you don't have to brave the fitness centre either – I know how intimidating it can be to walk into a changing room full of size-10 gym bunnies – but it is important to start moving your body somehow, even if your diet is going well or you don't need to lose weight. If you want to stay in shape for good, you're going to have to change your lifestyle and start using up those extra calories.

Exercise is also important if you simply want to stay supple, fit and healthy. And did I mention how great it can make you feel? I've never really understood why, but the more exercise I do, the more energy I have!

Staying in shape will make you happier, I promise. So many unfit women say that they are happy just the way they are; I've said it myself in the past. But having been at both ends of the scale, I now know what works for me.

'SO WHAT'S THE SECRET, I HEAR YOU CRY! WELL, FOR ME, IT'S DANCING ROUND MY HANDBAG… SORT OF!'

I never wanted to be skinny – well, not super-skinny anyway. I don't have four spare hours a day to spend in the gym and I've never wanted to look like Madonna. I see her and think, 'She's not having much fun'. And what's with the muscly arms? They're just scary!

No, I wanted to be a healthier weight and I wanted more energy, and with exercise I've achieved both. I'm probably fitter now than I've ever been in my adult life. My exercise regime has also had the added bonus of letting me set a good example to Ciara; starving then stuffing yourself again is not the kind of message a mother ought to pass on.

So what's the secret, I hear you cry! Well, for me, it's dancing round my handbag…sort of!

Doesn't every woman love to dance? Remember when you were younger, how you could dance all night and never once think of it as a chore? Dancing uses almost 300 calories an hour, making the body burn off fat so that you lose weight. It also raises your heart rate, strengthens your bones – warding off the brittle-bone disease osteoporosis – and improves your posture. It gives you long, lean muscles, makes you fitter and is very sexy if you can persuade your partner to do it with you.

As TV programmes such as *Strictly Come Dancing* and *Dancing on Ice* have shown, any sort of dancing is great for the body. But for me, the ultimate jiggling around has to be disco dancing, and that's what's been keeping me on the move for the past couple of years. You might prefer a tango or a sexy salsa; it doesn't really matter what you do, just do it, and do it regularly.

If you can, put aside between twenty minutes and an hour a day, whatever you can manage, and devote that time to yourself. In fact, my last DVD consists of four twenty-minute sections and, let's be honest, you'd be lying if you said you couldn't find a spare twenty minutes. I used to say that I had no time, but the truth is, there was always time for chocolate biscuits and Cadbury's Dairy Milk. Doing even a little bit of exercise is so much better than doing nothing; just think of the health benefits if nothing else. Now I find the time to exercise and I feel a trillion times better.

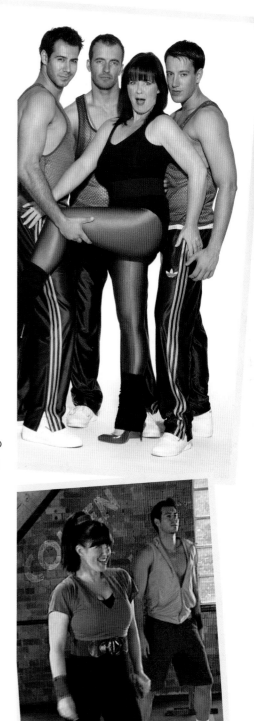

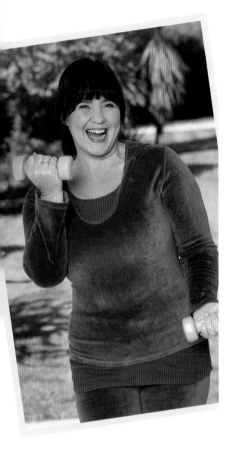

GETTING PHYSICAL

TO ENCOURAGE ME TO GET FIT, I WANTED A
WORKOUT THAT FELT LIKE FUN RATHER THAN EXERCISE.
THEN I MET MY FIRST PERSONAL TRAINER, MIKEY SMITH,
AND HE REALLY UNDERSTOOD WHAT I WAS AFTER.

We'd get together at my house in Cheshire and devise
routines based on the disco songs I love by all-time greats
like Gloria Gaynor, Rose Royce and Sister Sledge. We even
choreographed some routines to my own Nolan hits, such as
I'm in the Mood for Dancing, and this routine became
my fitness DVD *Disco Burn*.

Last year I needed some fresh motivation to help me
maintain my weight loss, so I devised a new DVD called *Let's
Get Physical*. With my new trainer, *GMTV*'s Deanne Berry, we
came up with four great new workouts, each of them only
twenty minutes long. It's still just dancing, but this time to all
my Eighties favourites, and the moves burn off the fat almost
without you noticing. When we recorded it I was really
conscious of the three rather attractive men dancing behind
me in the studio – I was glad my bum was five sizes smaller!

You can use *Let's Get Physical* or *Disco Burn* to get into
shape or you can simply follow these guidelines and then
invent your own routine. Remember, though, you have to
dance for long enough to raise your heartbeat and fast
enough so that it warms you up nicely. But whatever you do,
just get moving!

Get Moving in Eight Steps…

1 FIND A TIME THAT'S RIGHT FOR YOU. You may have to set the alarm half an hour earlier to find extra minutes, but choose a time that works for you and stick to it.

2 GET THE RIGHT EQUIPMENT. Invest in a pair of trainers and a tracksuit – if you have boobs like mine you also need a sports bra.

3 TELL YOURSELF THIS IS A REGULAR COMMITMENT. Ideally you want to exercise every day, but an hour just three times a week will make a huge difference.

4 DON'T LEAP INTO YOUR ROUTINE without first stretching and warming up. You don't want to hurt yourself by pulling a muscle.

5 IF YOUR FITNESS LEVELS ARE LOW, then start slowly and gradually increase the amount you can do.

6 AS YOU EXERCISE, THINK ABOUT IMPROVING YOUR POSTURE. This is your valuable time so you might as well get double the benefits. If you stand tall, push your shoulders back, pull your tummy in and squeeze your buttocks, you will burn even more calories, and your improved posture will make you look slimmer, too. If you are worried about your posture, you could think about doing a Pilates course, or just buy a good DVD. Pilates is brilliant for improving your posture, strengthening your core and toning your muscles. Even if you can't manage most exercises there will be a Pilates exercise that you can do – you can even practise pelvic floor exercises while you're watching telly!

7 THINK ABOUT WHICH PARTS OF YOUR BODY YOU WANT TO IMPROVE and introduce some specific toning exercises (see the end of the chapter). You want to burn calories, but it's also important to work on your problem areas.

8 WHEN YOU'VE COMPLETED YOUR ROUTINE, make sure you cool down with some stretches – that way tired muscles won't cramp.

Or Why Not Try...

If you have two left feet – and even then there's no reason why you can't enjoy a boogie in private – or you'd prefer to get out of the house to do your exercise, there are plenty of other easy ways to get moving. Here are five of my favourite activities. Every one of them will keep you fit without breaking the bank, causing you embarrassment or putting you in hospital.

● *Walking*

Number one in my book because it's absolutely free! We have two dogs and I love pulling on my boots, getting out into the fresh air and walking their little legs off. Try getting off the bus a few stops before your destination and walking the rest of the way; walk the kids to school, or just step out there and start getting to know your neighbourhood a little better - it's amazing what you see when you're not inside a car. Walking is great for your bones, your stress levels and your general fitness, and you'll burn off extra calories if your stride is quick enough. To get the best results, get to the point at which you feel you are about to break into a jog, then pull back slightly. Maintain that pace and aim to walk three or four miles an hour to feel the benefits.

> **CALORIE COUNTER**
> *= around 80 calories per mile or 280 calories an hour*

● *Housework and Gardening*

I can't pretend that cleaning the loo and scrubbing my patio doors are my favourite pastimes but sometimes, when the house is a tip and the garden looks like a jungle, there's nothing more satisfying than putting on some old clothes and really going for it. Sometimes I dance while I vacuum; other times I practise my squats and lunges while I trim the roses. And getting the old lawnmower out and giving the grass a good cut is a fantastic workout.

> **CALORIE COUNTER** = *around 200 calories an hour*

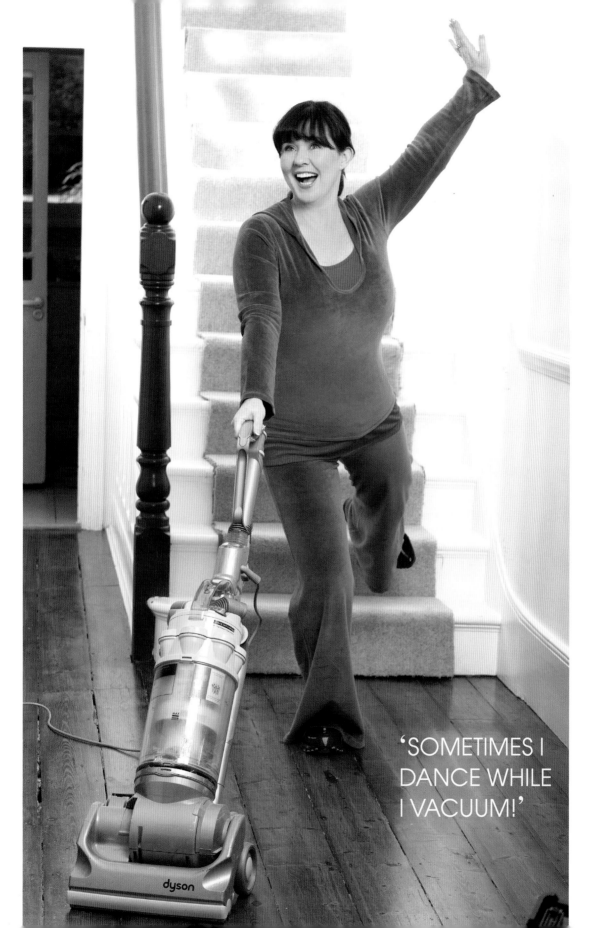

'SOMETIMES I DANCE WHILE I VACUUM!'

Swimming

I love swimming and it's a lot more pleasant these days than when I was a child and the local pools were freezing cold and cheerless. Swimming is not only a fantastic calorie burner, it's also a full-body workout, plus it's gentle on your joints because the water supports the body and doesn't put pressure on your bones and ligaments. Swimming regularly will improve your metabolism and help you de-stress after a busy day. It's not expensive either – most leisure centres will have deals for regular swimmers and you won't need to splash out on anything except a costume and a pair of goggles.

CALORIE COUNTER = *around 500 calories an hour*

Cycling

The beauty of cycling is that it doubles as exercise and transport: it can save you money on petrol or bus fares and give you a great workout at the same time. I can't quite believe it now, but in 2007 Ray and I cycled along the Nile to raise money for the Alzheimer's Society, the disease that took my lovely mum. We cycled more than fifty miles a day for five days and by the end of it I was knackered! It was a fantastic challenge and I'm glad we did it, but never again – I had blisters on my blisters and my shorts turned into cheese graters! Happily, you don't need to go to such lengths. Just get on your bike and you'll tone your legs, bottom and thighs and you won't put as much pressure on your knees, hips and ankles as you would when jogging. A good bicycle doesn't have to be expensive; keep an eye out for second-hand bargains in your local newspaper, but make sure all the gears and brakes are in good order. And please remember to wear a helmet.

CALORIE COUNTER = *around 550 calories an hour*

Ice Skating

I had to include skating because, as you see every year from the contestants on *Dancing on Ice*, it is brilliant for firming your thigh and calf muscles and tightening up

'ICE SKATING CAN BE A WONDERFUL WAY OF GETTING FIT. IT'S FUN, YOU CAN DO IT WITH THE KIDS AND EVERY LITTLE PROBLEM IN YOUR HEAD DISAPPEARS THE MOMENT YOU STEP ONTO THE ICE'

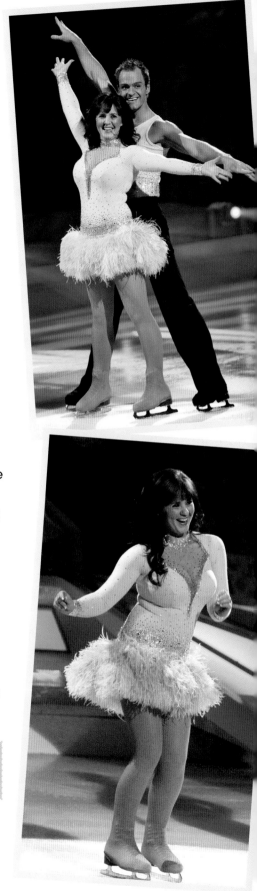

your bum. It's also a fantastic workout for your heart and lungs as the body has to work harder to maintain its temperature in the chilly conditions. That's not to say I loved every moment of my time on the show – in fact, some days I hated it, but assuming you're not going to be training to appear on live TV, dancing alongside Torvill and Dean, ice skating can be a wonderful way of getting fit. It's fun, you can do it with the kids and every little problem in your head disappears the moment you step onto the ice. Lots of towns have year-round indoor rinks, and more and more Christmas skating rinks seem to be popping up. When I was filming *Dancing on Ice Friday* with the lovely Ben Shephard, every time I saw one of the contestants on their bum on the ice I thanked my lucky stars that it wasn't me. Skating is fantastic exercise, and if you take it easy you should even avoid the accident and emergency department!

CALORIE COUNTER
= *around 500 calories an hour*

No Time for a Workout?

Yes, yes, I used to say that too. If you really can't find an extra half-hour for yourself, then there are still ways you can fit exercise into your life. The trick is to remember that you are no longer a couch potato, that you want to change your life and that given the choice you will never again opt for the lazy way of doing things.

- It's an obvious one this, but if you're at work or in a department store, take the stairs rather than the lift, or walk up the escalators and then back down again.

- Hide the TV remote control. Remember how we actually used to stand up and use our legs when we wanted to change channel? Why not go back to those good old days and use up a few calories?

- Sack the window cleaner and do it yourself. OK, so it might be a bit tricky doing the top floors, but you could at least do the ground-floor windows and the insides. It's a great exercise for getting rid of those bingo wings.

- If you spend your Saturdays or Sundays standing on the sideline watching your kids or partner taking part in a football or rugby match, then you're missing an ideal opportunity to exercise. Don't just stand there, stride around the field while you watch.

- Take the family indoor bowling…but stay away from the bar and the popcorn.

- Every time you speak on the telephone, stand up and walk around. Tell yourself you're not allowed to sit down while you're on the phone. You'll walk off a few calories and you might even reduce your phone bills.

- Use the kids' games console to get fit. You'll obviously have to fork out for the console and game, but if your family are already spending lots of time on the PlayStation, X-Box or Wii, they might as well join you in a bit of gaming exercise. You can buy interactive games that get you moving for all three types of console, although Nintendo's Wii Fit is undoubtedly the pick of the bunch. Just make sure you don't end up playing a stationary game where the only part of your body that gets exercised are your thumbs!

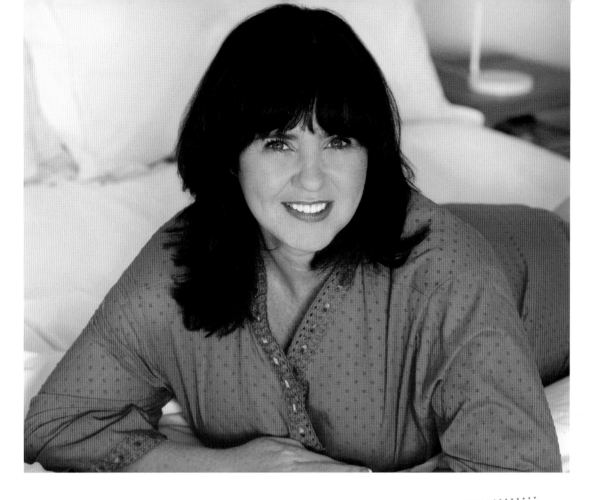

The Best Exercise of Them All!

Why is it that most naughty things are bad for us: chocolate HobNobs, a nice glass of wine, bacon sandwiches on white bread with lots of butter. It's not fair, is it? But there is one naughty activity that's very good for us indeed. Yep, sex!

Experts say that thirty minutes – erm, that's right, thirty minutes, sorry about that – of sex burns around 100 calories and the exercise helps keep you happy and flexible. Sex can also cure headaches, reduce stress and improve circulation, not to mention help you sleep.

So the next time the old man starts getting frisky, don't pretend to be asleep, think of the calories!

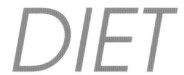

DIET

FOR EXERCISE TO BE SUCCESSFUL, IT MUST BE COMBINED WITH HEALTHY EATING. AND WHETHER OR NOT YOU HAVE WEIGHT TO LOSE, IT'S IMPORTANT TO HAVE A GOOD DIET IN ORDER TO STAY FIT, HEALTHY AND HAPPY.

Remember, as we've already seen in earlier chapters, food plays an enormous part in how we look. Just think about how bad your skin looks when you've overdone the chocolate, or how sluggish you feel if you've been living off junk food for a while.

I think the word 'diet' is a killer when you're trying to lose weight. Don't think of it as 'being good' or as an eating regime you're only going to do until you get into that size-12 dress. Tell yourself this is the start of a new you and the beginning of the rest of your life. Don't think of it as 'going without' but as 'healthy eating' and as something you're doing because you are now taking better care of yourself and because you deserve it! You'll find you can still have treats if you're eating healthily most of the time.

I'm afraid my absolute favourite foods are those that are really bad for you: Italian dishes with rich cheesy sauces, bread and chocolate. It seems I'm drawn to the naughtiest things in life. I've tried total deprivation. I've cut out all these things from my diet before, but you know what, they always sneak back in, and by then I want them tenfold. Just one moment of weakness and, as if by magic, there's a family-sized pizza box in my hand.

These days I try to trick my brain into behaving. I never say never, I just say I'll have it later. And if friends come round to the house and suggest ordering a Chinese, I say yes – I just don't say yes four times a week!

The experts I've worked with on my DVDs have shown me how to spread my calorie intake over the day. They explained that by grazing constantly rather than stuffing myself when I'm starving, I will be more in control of what I eat. Now, because I'm never really hungry and my energy levels don't dip, I'm less tempted to dive into the biscuit tin.

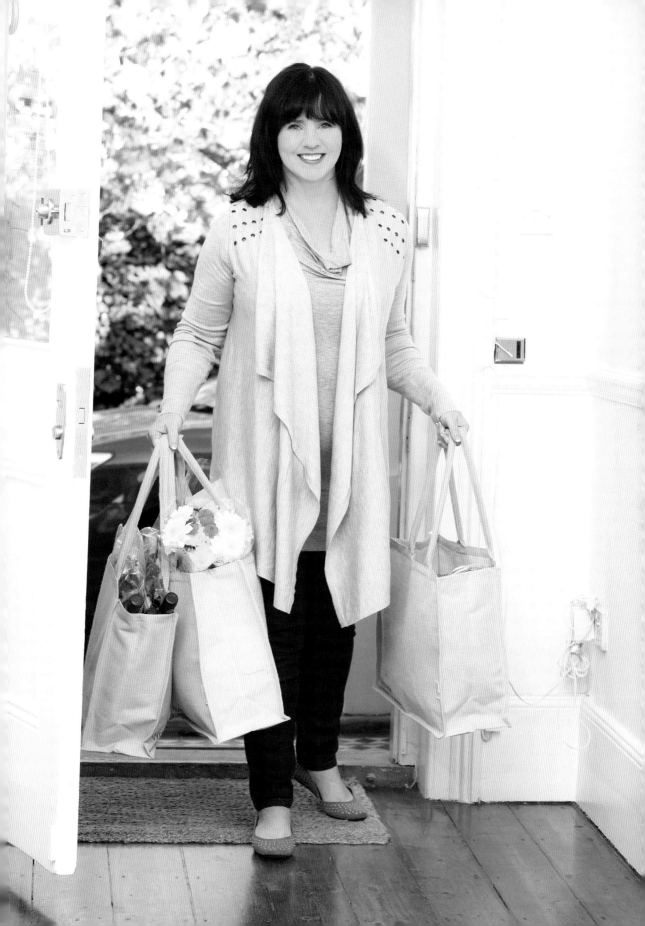

I try to fit five or six meals into my day: breakfast, a morning snack, lunch, an afternoon snack, evening meal and then an evening snack. It sounds like a lot, but it's all the right kind of food.

Daily Menu

• Breakfast

Fruit with natural yoghurt, porridge (no sugar) or a low-calorie breakfast cereal.

• Mid-Morning Snack

Health bar, an apple or an orange, or a fruit smoothie.

• Lunch

Salad with lean meat, tuna or low-fat cottage cheese. Don't be tempted to use ordinary mayonnaise or salad dressing as they can be really high in calories. Use a low-calorie option or make your own dressing with lemon juice. If you don't fancy salad, try low-fat hummus on an oatcake or rice cake.

• Afternoon Snack

Fruit, chopped-up raw veg, for example red peppers or carrots, or low-fat yoghurt with a handful of nuts.

• Evening Meal

Go for lean meat or fish, plenty of vegetables or salad and not too many potatoes or too much pasta. If you can, it's best to steer clear of bad carbohydrates, such as white bread or pasta, this late in the day. You may not have eaten wholegrain pasta before, but why not give it a try? You'll get used to it really quickly and after a short while you'll hardly notice the difference. Good carbs are found in wholemeal foods, fruit and vegetables, and are higher in fibre so they make you feel fuller for longer. If you want to eat carbohydrates in the evening, good carbs are the ones to choose, such as brown rice, wholegrain pasta, quinoa, beans and lentils.

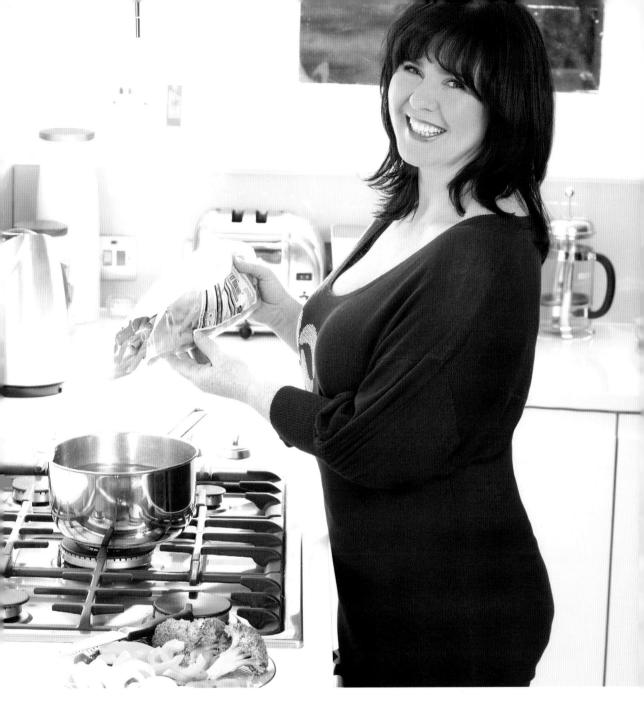

● *Evening Snack*

Have a healthy evening snack planned well in advance so that you're not left gazing longingly at the biscuit tin. I often have crispbreads, fruit or a glass of milk, and if I'm feeling naughty I'll either have a low-fat instant hot-chocolate drink or a slice of malt loaf – without any butter!

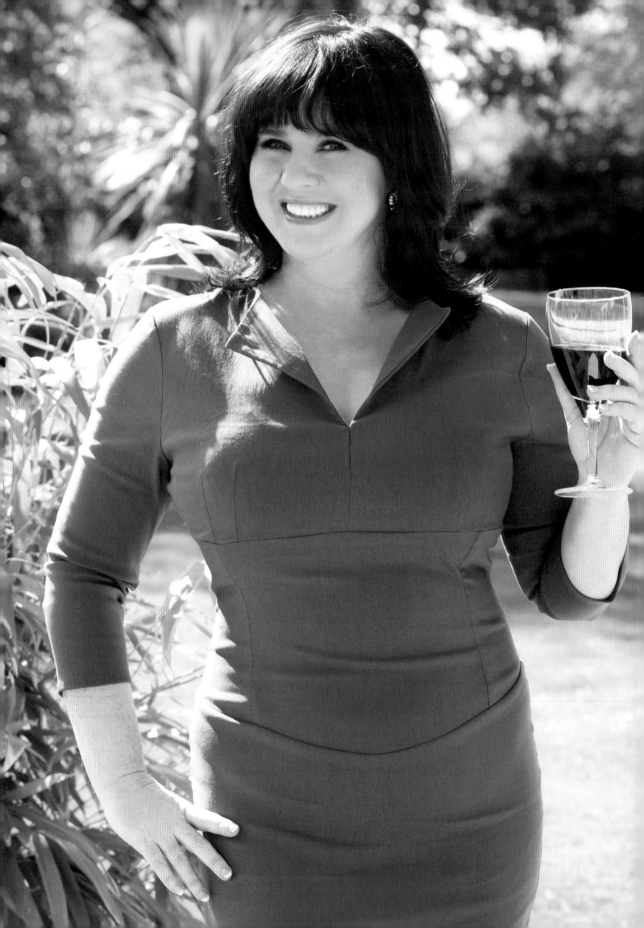

Make Mine a Pint ... (of Water!)

I'm not really a big drinker (honestly, I'm a really cheap date!) so it isn't difficult for me to say no to a tipple. But for lots of people alcohol is the last thing they want to give up. I'm not saying you can never drink again, but if you do want to get in shape you need to control your alcohol intake. It's not a bad idea for health reasons, too.

Here's the calorie countdown for some popular tipples. Next time you fancy a cheeky one, it might be useful to know which drinks are saintly and which are sinful!

- Half a pint of bitter: 91 calories
- Standard glass of red wine (175ml): 119 calories
- Half a pint of lager: 122 calories
- Standard glass of white wine (175ml): 130 calories
- Standard glass of sparkling white wine: 131 calories
- Standard measure of Baileys (50ml): 175 calories
- Bottle of alcopop: 198 calories

Of course, the drink with absolutely no calories is water. Not the most fun a girl can have on a night out, granted, but a long glass of sparkling water with lots of ice and a slice of lime can be really refreshing. Remember to drink plenty of ordinary still water throughout the day, too, as it will help fill you up and keep you hydrated.

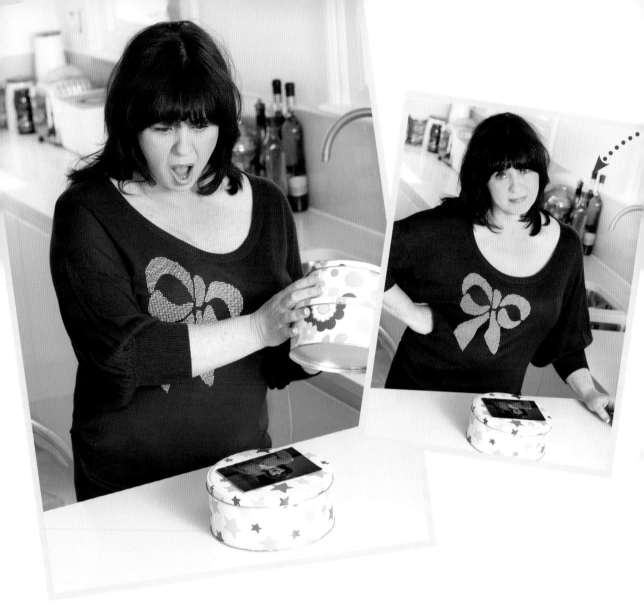

Mrs Motivator

I'm not pretending any of this is easy. Believe me, there were lots of times when I well and truly fell off the wagon – sometimes with a Wagon Wheel biscuit in my hand! My family used to tease me about my lack of willpower – I was a notorious 'start tomorrow' dieter. To be honest, I'm not really sure how I finally managed to crack it. I'd be fibbing if I said I hadn't put a few pounds back on, but it's all about finding a comfortable, healthy weight without returning to yo-yo dieting. I don't know if this is 'me' for life but so far, so good. What I do know is that it's vital to have some golden motivators, and these were the ten commandments I stuck to. If I can do it, then so can you…

1 PLACE YOUR WORST 'FAT' PHOTO SOMEWHERE YOU CAN SEE IT whenever you're tempted to go off the rails – you could even sticky-tape it to the biscuit tin.

2 GIVE YOURSELF A GOOD INCENTIVE. Mine was wanting to look my best for my wedding.

3 NEVER GO HUNGRY OR MISS A MEAL. If you're not hungry you won't be tempted by rubbish. Eat three main meals and fill up on low-calorie foods.

4 DON'T DEPRIVE YOURSELF. I never say, 'I won't,' I just say, 'I won't now – maybe later,' and usually the urge passes. If I can't shake off that desire for a biscuit then I have one; I just don't eat the entire packet!

5 DON'T PANIC IF YOU DO PUT ON SOME WEIGHT – just catch it before it gets out of hand. I've learned that it's far easier to shift half a stone than get rid of five.

6 START YOUR DAY AS A WINNER. Eat a healthy breakfast, take the dog for a walk, make yourself a smoothie – do something positive and the rest of the day should follow suit.

7 GET RID OF YOUR 'FAT' CLOTHES. Every time I went down a dress size I took any clothes that were too big for me to the charity shop. Otherwise it's easy to drift back into your comfy tracksuit bottoms.

8 REMEMBER WHO'S IN CHARGE. Don't let your life be dictated by food; stay in control and don't be bullied by a pizza or a packet of custard creams.

9 EAT TO LIVE, DON'T LIVE TO EAT. Sharing a meal with your friends and family is a pleasure, but try to remember what's really important – here's a clue: it's usually sitting opposite you, not on your plate.

10 DON'T LOSE WEIGHT FOR ANYONE OTHER THAN YOURSELF. The truth is, no one cares what your dress size is as much as you do. Don't listen to those who try to lead you astray; think of your new healthy body as a gift to yourself and make sure you deliver!

HELP YOURSELF FOR FREE

NOW THAT I'VE HOPEFULLY GOT YOU BOPPING AROUND YOUR LIVING ROOM, IT'S TIME TO THINK ABOUT SPECIFIC EXERCISES TO TACKLE THOSE PROBLEM AREAS WE ALL HAVE.

I'm quite lucky that my body is relatively in proportion. Even when I was very overweight, I was heavier all over, and I seem to have lost weight from everywhere, rather than from just my boobs or bum. We all have areas of our bodies that we like more than others. My legs weren't too bad, but I hated my upper arms. Losing weight through diet and aerobic exercise, such as dancing, will help trim these hated areas, but to really tackle the problem you need to tighten the muscles around them.

Don't panic, you won't need expensive gym memberships or fancy weights. To be honest, when I train I still use bottles of water and tins of beans as weights, and you can do the same. Give it a go and get trim without spending a penny.'

'WHEN I TRAIN I STILL USE BOTTLES OF WATER AND TINS OF BEANS AS WEIGHTS…GET TRIM WITHOUT SPENDING A PENNY'

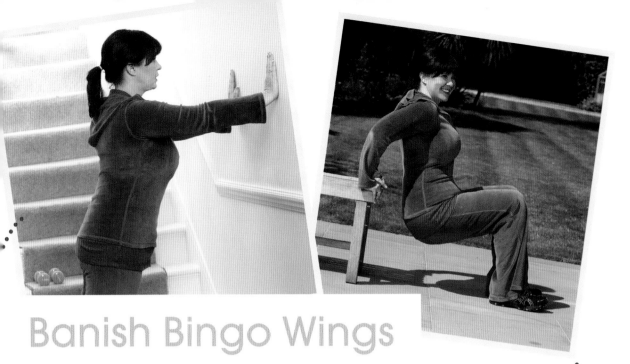

Banish Bingo Wings

Squeeze this set of 100 REPETITIONS into your routine as often as you can and you'll soon firm up your wobbly upper arms.

● Stand facing a wall, with your feet about a foot from the skirting board and your hands flat against it. Keeping your back straight, touch your nose to the wall, then push yourself back until your arms are fully extended.
REPEAT TWENTY-FIVE TIMES

● Sit on a dining-room or kitchen chair (without arms – the chair, not you), put your feet flat on the floor about a foot in front of you and slide your bottom to the front of the seat. Grip the sides of the chair and, using your arms for support, slide your bottom off the seat. Bend your elbows to lower your bottom a few inches, then straighten them to pull your bottom back onto the chair. Keep your shoulders straight and your neck long.
REPEAT TWENTY-FIVE TIMES

● Holding a tin of beans in each hand, start with your arms down by your sides and then bend your elbows, bringing your hands to your shoulders.
REPEAT TWENTY-FIVE TIMES

● Next, bend your arms at the elbows and raise the tins of beans into the air until your arms are straight.
REPEAT TWENTY-FIVE TIMES

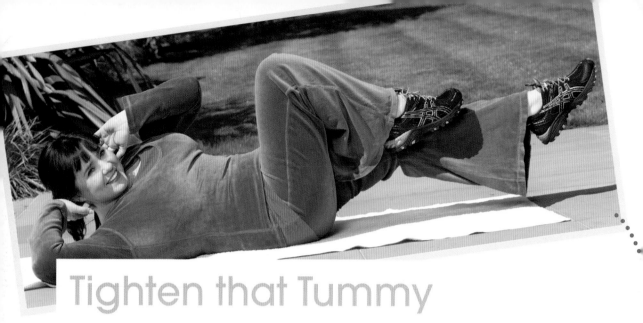

Tighten that Tummy

You don't have to torture yourself with punishing full crunches to get a trimmer tummy;
just repeat these gentle exercises regularly and you'll see an improvement:

● Lie down and press your lower back into the floor. Bend your knees and bring
them up to your chest. Place your hands behind your ears. Now start cycling
with your legs, straightening one leg at a time. Raise your shoulders and touch
your elbow to the opposite bent knee as you do so. Work from your waist
and don't pull your neck.
REPEAT TWENTY-FIVE TIMES

● Lie on the floor and tuck your toes under your bed or the sofa – depending on
which room you are using – then gently raise your head and shoulders, keeping
your neck long and straight. Keep your arms straight in front of you and try to
slide them down to your knees.
REPEAT TWENTY-FIVE TIMES

● Lie on your back with your legs bent and your feet flat on the floor about a
foot apart. Place your hands across your chest and slowly lift your head and
shoulders off the floor, then lower them back down again.
REPEAT TWENTY-FIVE TIMES

● Lie on the floor and raise your legs into the air, making a 90-degree angle at
the hips. Use your tummy muscles to push your feet towards the ceiling as far as
you can.
REPEAT TWENTY-FIVE TIMES

No More Love Handles

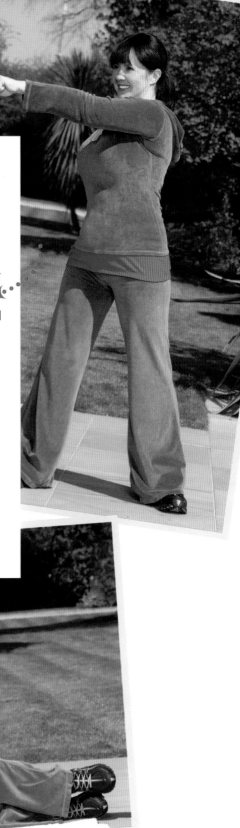

When I was bigger, I certainly never loved those little rolls of fat that hung over the sides of my jeans. Tummy exercises are fantastic for the whole of your middle, but if you want to strengthen your side abs and remove your muffin top, try these exercises:

● Stand with your feet about a foot apart and twist your upper body to the left, keeping your hips facing the front. As you twist, punch your right hand out diagonally over your left toes, keeping your arm horizontal. Now twist to the right and punch your left hand over your right toes. Feel the twist in your waist.

REPEAT FIFTY TIMES

● Lie on your side and raise your upper body with your elbow and lower arm supporting you. Keep your body straight and your neck long. Using your tummy muscles, raise your hips and hold yourself off the floor for twenty-five seconds. Change sides and hold for another twenty-five seconds.

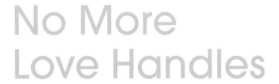

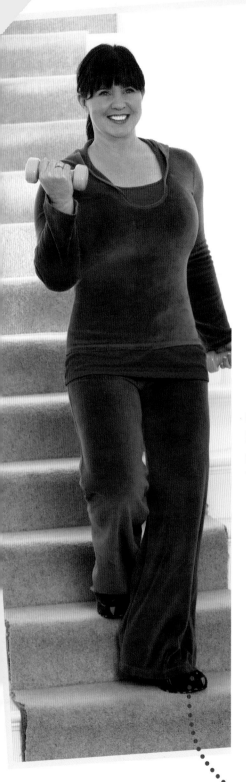

'SOME OF MY *DANCING ON ICE* COSTUMES LEFT VERY LITTLE TO THE IMAGINATION'

Cheeky Bottom Exercises

Some of my *Dancing on Ice* costumes left very little to the imagination, so I was glad I'd worked so hard to reduce the size of my backside before I had to squeeze into them! These exercises are great for firming your buttocks:

- Squeeze the cheeks of your bottom in and out – no one even needs to know!
  REPEAT FIFTY TIMES WHEN YOU REMEMBER

- You'd usually do this one on a step in the gym, but you could use your bottom stair. Stand with your back to the staircase and, keeping your hips straight, flex your right foot and lower your heel as far as you can to the floor. Bring it back onto the step and do the same for your left foot.
  REPEAT FIFTY TIMES IN TOTAL

- Walk up and down the stairs twenty-five times. If you can't manage this, start with ten sets and work your way up.

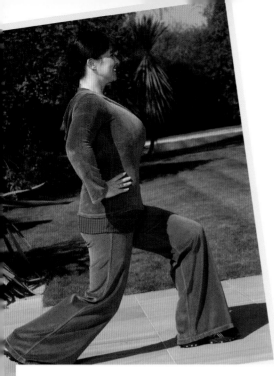

The Thigh's the Limit!

I used to be really conscious of my wobbly thighs. If you need to firm up your inner thighs, these are the exercises for you:

- Sit on the floor with your legs stretched out and a dining chair in front of you. Place your feet either side of the legs, then squeeze your legs together so you can feel the muscles of your inner thighs working. Hold for five seconds and relax.
REPEAT TWENTY-FIVE TIMES

- There is such a thing as a free lunge! Stand up straight and put one foot forward as far as is comfortable. Bend your knees and dip as low as you can without your back knee touching the floor. Your front knee should be in line with your toes. Hold this position for twenty-five seconds, then change to the other side.
REPEAT TEN TIMES ON EACH SIDE

- Lie on your right side so your head's in line with your shoulders, hips and feet. Bend your left (top) leg and bring it in front of you so your thigh is at a right angle to your body. Next, lift your right (lower) leg off the floor. Hold this position for twenty-five seconds, then relax and lift again.
REPEAT FOUR TIMES ON EACH SIDE

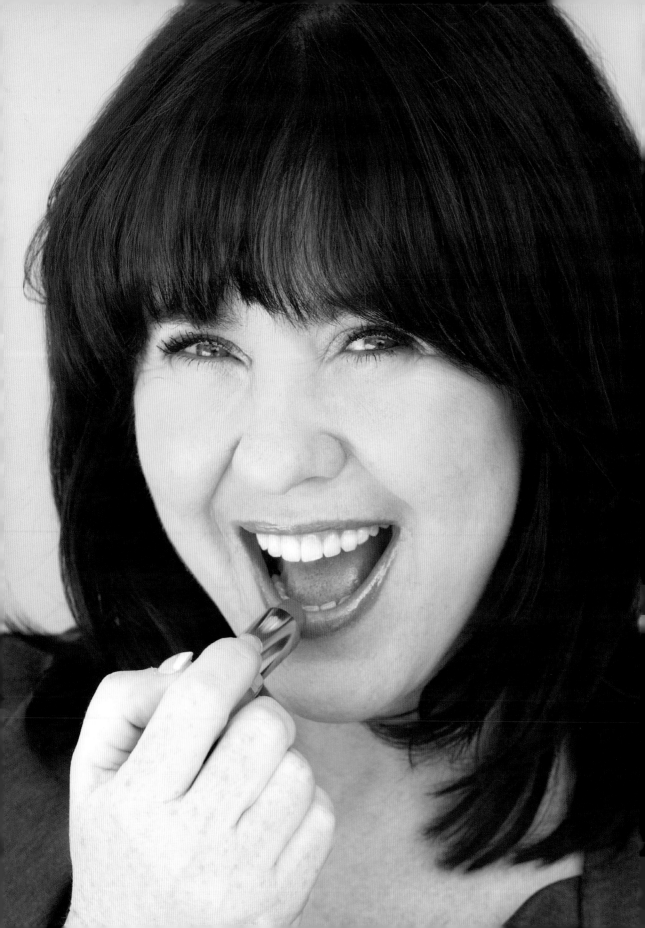

CHAPTER 7

Gotta pull myself together...

LOOKING YOUR BEST

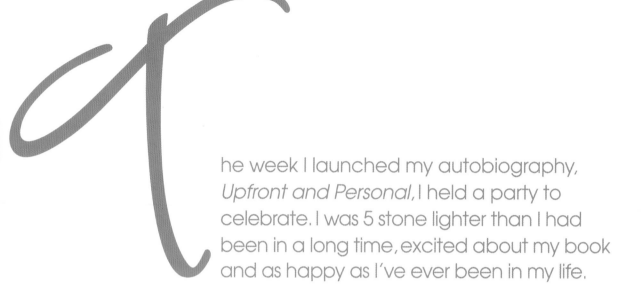

The week I launched my autobiography, *Upfront and Personal*, I held a party to celebrate. I was 5 stone lighter than I had been in a long time, excited about my book and as happy as I've ever been in my life.

I decided I was going to wear something amazing and, after a lot of soul-searching, I opted for a pair of black wet-look leggings, a sparkly suit jacket and skyscraper heels.

I felt fantastic that night. Ray told me I looked beautiful and, as I arrived at the do, I happily posed for photographs knowing that I'd be in the newspapers the next morning.

Oh. My. God. What a fall from grace. The fashion gestapo had a field day and I was slaughtered for dressing too young. One male journalist even sneered, 'We're glad she's not our mum.' What a nasty thing to say!

I have a real fear of appearing in those awful worst-dressed sections of newspapers and magazines, and for a moment I was mortified. I hated people thinking I was mutton dressed as lamb and that I'd forgotten I was really a forty-four-year-old mum of three. But then I gave myself a talking-to. I reminded myself that I hadn't gone out flashing my bum in a micro-mini skirt; neither had I worn a leather bra top and shown everyone my not-so-washboard stomach.

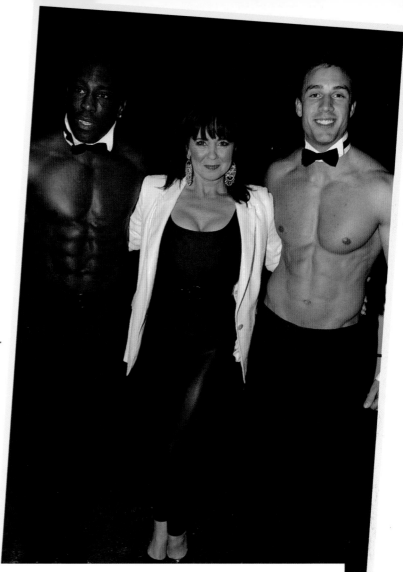

> **'A SPARKLY JACKET AND A PAIR OF WET-LOOK LEGGINGS CAN GIVE YOU A BOOST YOU CAN'T BOTTLE'**

I'd chosen my clothes carefully, mixing the funky leggings with a sophisticated grown-up jacket. And what's more, my husband had absolutely loved my outfit. He thought I looked wonderful and, because I trust him, his opinion is more important to me than that of any fashion critic or bitchy columnist.

The moral of the story is that, in the end, I didn't get upset and burn the leggings. I might not wear them to another showbiz party in a hurry, but I still pull them on from time to time and they still make me feel wonderful.

And that's the power of fashion. A beautiful dress can make you feel a trillion dollars. Killer heels can give you confidence as well as inches. And a sparkly jacket and a pair of wet-look leggings can give you a boost you can't bottle.

'I'VE GOT TO THE AGE WHERE I KNOW WHAT SUITS ME, AND WITH A LITTLE GUIDANCE YOU CAN KNOW WHAT SUITS YOU, TOO'

The trick is knowing your body shape, discovering what suits you and not dressing too young – or too old – for your age.

You don't need to spend a fortune on clothes – my sparkly jacket was from a bargain-basement high-street store – nor do you need to be on the cutting edge of fashion: just because something's ultra trendy doesn't mean it's going to suit you. You don't even need to have a model figure to look good. Dressing well is about putting some thought into your wardrobe, not living exclusively in leggings and baggy T-shirts and not being dictated to by the fashion police.

In my job, I'm lucky enough to work with stylists who have years of experience dressing women. But sometimes the stylist gets it wrong and they'll put me in clothes that are too young, or even sometimes clothes that make me look like my granny.

I now know that fitted clothes suit me best, such as lovely tailored trousers and dresses that pull me in and emphasise my boobs and waist. I don't feel comfortable flashing my breasts too much – a little cleavage is fine, but I feel like Katie Price if I go too low – and I've learned I feel better if the tops of my arms are covered. I don't mind the shape of my legs, but I feel too pale to go without tights or to wear skirts that are too short.

Having lost some weight, I want to show off my figure, but without screaming, 'Look at me!' I've got to the age where I know what suits me, and with a little guidance you can know what suits you, too.

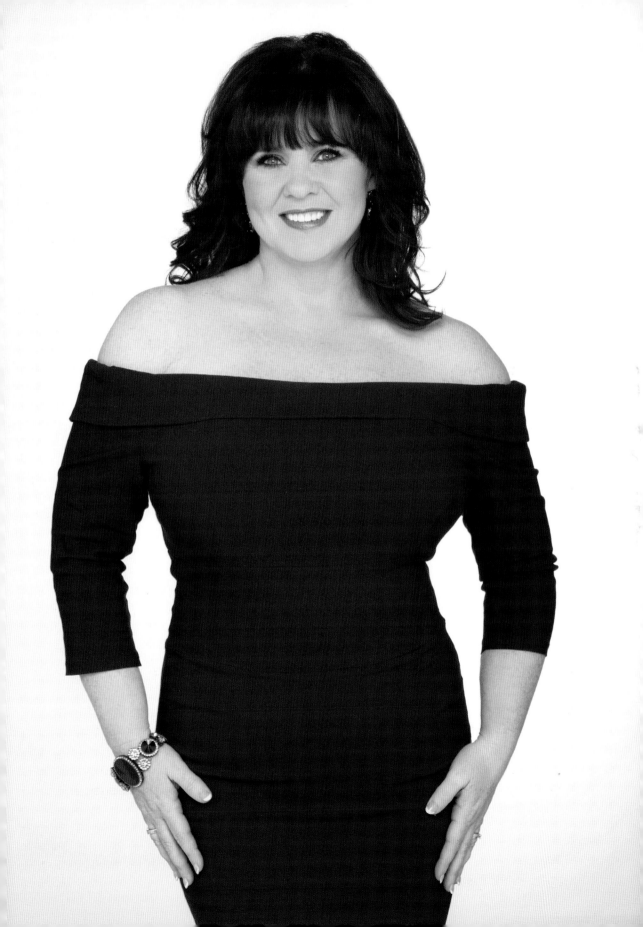

ACT YOUR AGE

IT'S DIFFICULT GETTING THE AGE THING RIGHT BECAUSE ALTHOUGH I'M IN MY MID-FORTIES, I DON'T FEEL ANY DIFFERENT THAN WHEN I WAS TWENTY. MIND YOU, I'D DEFINITELY GET SLAUGHTERED IN THE PRESS IF I WENT OUT IN SOME OF THE OUTFITS I WORE AS A GIRL OUT ON THE TOWN IN BLACKPOOL!

There is so much choice out there, but you have to be really honest with yourself. Even if you have a washboard stomach, should you be flashing it to all and sundry if you're not in your twenties or thirties? And although these days I could possibly just about crowbar myself into a tiny slip of a dress, would I feel comfortable?

The truth is that by dressing too young you actually make yourself look older. Wear a bra top and hipsters with your belly showing and you will look every one of your forty-four years. But there's no need to dress older than your age either. Some women say they can't wear trainers and jeans because they're, say, fifty. I say, you're fifty, not dead!

Take a good hard look in your wardrobe. Is it full of expensive mistakes? Do you need a makeover? If you're like me you might dread the thought of clothes shopping. I can almost hear the excuses from here: I haven't got time; I can't afford to; I'm hopeless at choosing clothes for myself; it doesn't matter what I wear.

The truth is, though, it does matter what you wear, even if it's just a pair of jeans that fit you fantastically. You may be able to fool yourself – and everybody else – that it doesn't, but just remember how good you felt the last time you wore an outfit that made you look great. But please don't panic; there are some simple rules, and together we'll learn how to follow them so that your clothes show off your best bits and help disguise the rest.

SHAPING UP

AS WE'VE ALREADY LEARNED, THERE ARE FOUR MAIN BODY SHAPES: **PEAR**, **APPLE**, **HOURGLASS** AND **ATHLETIC**. CERTAIN TYPES OF CLOTHES WILL SUIT YOUR SHAPE; IT'S JUST A CASE OF KNOWING WHERE YOU FIT IN.

Pear

Your upper body is smaller than your hips, thighs and bottom, so you need to emphasise your top half. You'll also look great if you draw attention to your delicate shoulders and arms.

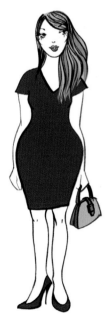

• Dos and Don'ts

DO: Wear darker clothes on the bottom half of your body.

DON'T: Wear tops that end around your hips and draw the eye to your widest part.

DO: Wear three-quarter-length sleeves that take the eye to waist height.

DON'T: Wear trousers and skirts with pleats or gathers or that are made from bulky material.

DO: Wear straight or wide-legged jeans or trousers.

DON'T: Wear patterns on your bottom half.

DO: Wear halterneck or strapless dresses and tops to widen your shoulders.

DON'T: Wear horizontal stripes on your lower half – keep them for tops only.

DO: Wear skirts with asymmetric hemlines.

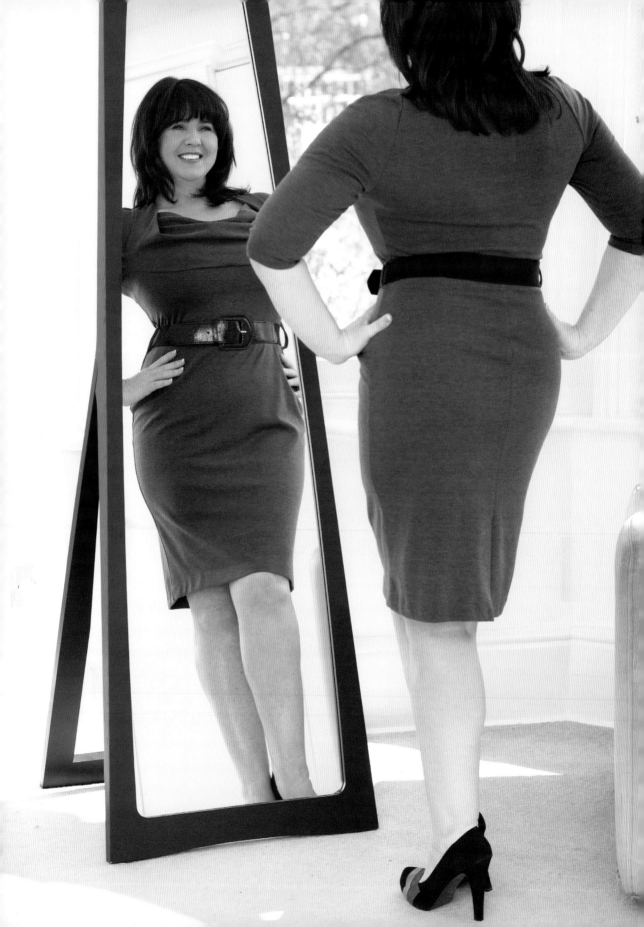

Apple

Your widest part is your middle and you have little waist definition, so you need to draw the eye to your shapely boobs and great legs.

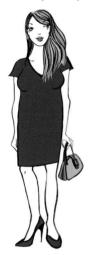

● *Dos and Don'ts*

DO: Wear above-the-knee skirts to show off your legs.
DON'T: Wear wide belts or skirts with gathered waists.
DO: Wear tunic-shaped tops that slide over your hips.
DON'T: Wear wide-legged trousers.
DO: Wear skirts and trousers that fasten at the side.
DON'T: Wear tight-fitting pencil skirts.
DO: Wear tops that fit around the boobs, then flare out over the stomach.
DON'T: Wear tops with high necklines – show off your cleavage and draw the eye away from your waistline.

Hourglass

With your nipped-in waist and curvy top and bottom, this is an easier shape to dress. Show off the bits that go in and out and you'll be on to a winner.

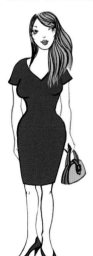

● *Dos and Don'ts*

DO: Wear belted wrap dresses to show off your waist.
DON'T: Wear boxy, shapeless tunics or dresses that will make you look bigger all over.
DO: Wear a bra that fits properly. Don't be afraid to show off the shape of your boobs, but make sure they look their best.
DON'T: Wear thick belts – you want to lengthen your body, not cut it in two.
DO: Wear tops that finish at the waist.
DON'T: Wear anything that is too baggy.
DO: Wear on- or below-the-knee skirts as they will lengthen your body.
DON'T: Wear tops with ruffles or fussy detail around the cleavage.

'THE TRUTH IS, THOUGH, IT DOES MATTER WHAT YOU WEAR, EVEN IF IT'S JUST A PAIR OF JEANS THAT FIT YOU FANTASTICALLY. YOU MAY BE ABLE TO FOOL YOURSELF – AND EVERYBODY ELSE – THAT IT DOESN'T, BUT JUST REMEMBER HOW GOOD YOU FELT THE LAST TIME YOU WORE AN OUTFIT THAT MADE YOU LOOK GREAT'

Athletic

Because you go straight up and down you can carry off most styles, but you need to choose clothes that emphasise your feminine side.

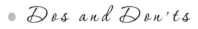 *Dos and Don'ts*

DO: Wear dresses with frills and ruffles to make you appear more shapely.

DON'T: Wear pencil skirts or very fitted dresses that show off every curve you don't have.

DO: Wear skinny jeans and tight-fitting trousers to emphasise your fantastic legs.

DON'T: Wear outfits that are all one colour: you should break up your shape with different patterns and shades.

DO: Wear tops that flare out at the waist to give the illusion of curves.

DON'T: Wear clothes that are too masculine – and don't forget to accessorise with pretty, girly jewellery.

DO: Wear belts over jumpers, cardigans and coats.

IF YOU HAVE...

Little Legs

Not everyone is in proportion and it can be a real pain if you have a long body but short legs. I don't mind the shape of my legs, but it would be wonderful if they were a few inches longer.

HERE ARE A FEW TIPS IF YOU WANT TO LOOK LEGGY:

- Always wear heels. It's not very practical to toddle about in stilettos all the time, but even a smaller heel will make your legs look longer and give extra height.

- Don't wear hipster jeans. Try jeans with a waist.

- Stay away from long jackets and shirts and instead choose fitted tops that finish at your waist.

- Look for high-waisted skirts, or those dresses that appear to be a top and high-waisted pencil skirt.

Big Boobs

It's true that the grass is always greener on the other side of the fence, and some of my girlfriends are very jealous of my well-endowed chest. But my big boobs have, in some ways, been the bane of my life. They started growing when I was thirteen years old and it feels they haven't stopped since! Even when I was at my slimmest they remained a 36FF – not that Ray was complaining. Sometimes I moan and ask him, 'Do my boobs look big in this?' He just laughs and says, 'Coleen, your boobs *are* big!'

- Make sure you wear a well-fitted bra (more on this later in the chapter).

- Don't try to hide them in baggy tops: you will only look bigger. Stick to fitted tops with a scooped or V-neck and wear a longer-length jacket or cardigan over the fitted top.

- Spend more money on your top half than your bottom. When finances are limited you might find a beautifully cut top is more of a friend than an expensive pair of jeans.

- Go for empire-line dresses or tops – fitted around the bust and flaring out below – as this seems to balance the boobs somehow.

- If all else fails, be proud and love them!

No Boobs

Like I said, the grass is always greener, and there have been many times in my life when I've wished I had a smaller chest. Most flat-chested women wouldn't agree with me, though, and many search for ways to boost their assets. Just look at the number of ladies having boob jobs these days.

HERE ARE A FEW SIMPLE WAYS TO GET OUT IN FRONT:

- The obvious saviour for smaller girls is the bra that gives you extra inches. A padded bra has pre-made cups that will make your boobs look bigger than they really are, while a push-up bra will give you a better cleavage. You could try slipping a couple of 'chicken fillets' into your bra – these are often made of silicone and sit inside your underwear to make you a few cup sizes larger.

- Wear shirts in solid, bright colours, or tops with horizontal stripes. Button-up shirts and T-shirts will enhance your boobs – just leave the top few buttons undone. Tops or dresses with a high neckline will make your boobs appear larger too.

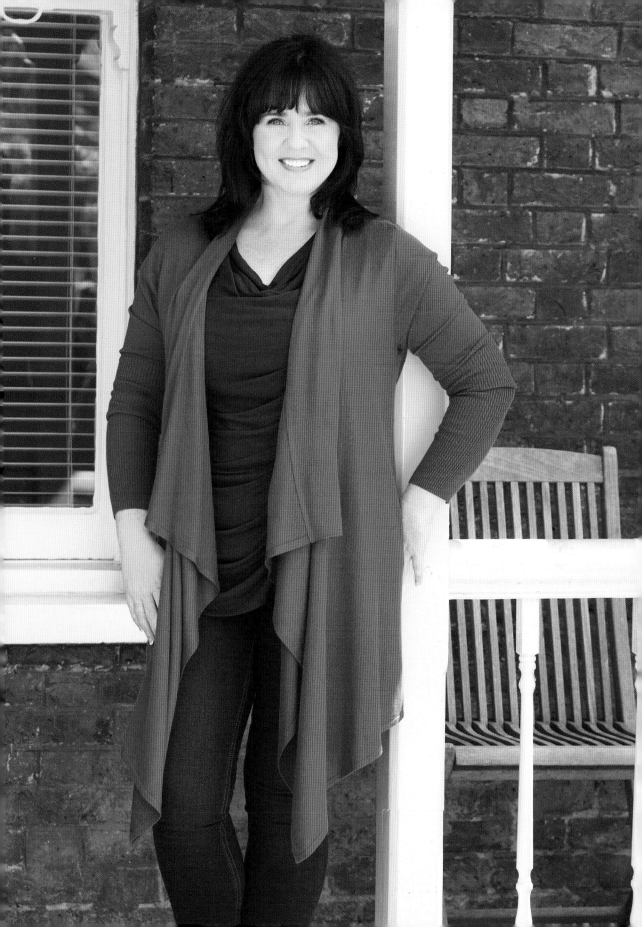

DRESS YOURSELF SLIM

I CAN LOOK TWO DRESS SIZES BIGGER JUST BY WEARING THE WRONG CLOTHES. BUT THE GOOD NEWS IS THAT WHEN I CHOOSE THE RIGHT COLOURS, FABRICS AND DESIGNS, I CAN SHRINK OVERNIGHT!

Size

The first and most important rule to remember is this: wear the correct size clothes. It's no good wishing you were the size 12 you used to be and squeezing into your old clothes regardless. And you should never wear clothes that are too baggy on you in a bid to hide your lumps and bumps. You will look slimmer if your dress or trousers aren't straining at the seams, and more streamlined if you don't look like you're drowning in your own clothes.

Line

The experts say never use pockets as they spoil the line of your clothes and make you look bigger. As a mum I know it's tempting to stuff half a box of tissues into your coat in case of emergencies, but do try not to. You could even sew them up to resist temptation!

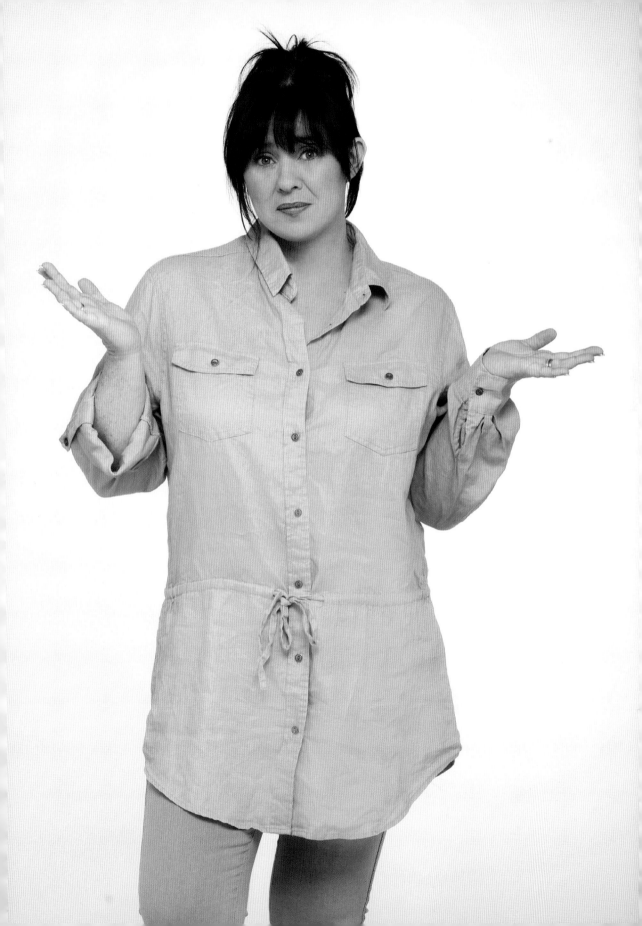

Colour

I don't care what the style queens on the telly say, black definitely makes me feel and look slimmer. It can be a bit boring, though, and for those with pale skin, like me, there is the danger you'll look washed out. Sticking to a single colour is a good trick, however, so why not experiment with other colours. You could try navy, grey or something a little brighter like a deep purple or red. Oh, and never wear colours on your bottom half that are lighter than those on the top.

Shape

You want to accentuate the tiniest parts of your body and disguise the bits you're embarrassed about. If you have a small waist, then cinch it in with a belt. If you hate your arms, then wear a three-quarter-length sleeve so the eye goes to your slim wrists. And if you have pretty ankles, don't cover them up.

Print

I've read all kinds of rules that say if you are bigger you shouldn't wear this or that stripe, or that you should steer clear of patterns all together. I don't think you necessarily have to do that, but I do find that the larger the print, the larger I feel. So if you don't want to keep it plain, make sure the pattern is small and delicate.

Extras

● *Accessories*

Strangely, the opposite is true for jewellery and handbags. Tiny bags and chains won't do you any favours, so go for chunky necklaces and beads, extravagant earrings and huge bags as they will make you look smaller.

● *Underwear*

Even though I've lost some weight, I'm still addicted to my Bridget Jones knickers. They ain't pretty, but they suck me in in all the right places.

Control pants are brilliant for a
quick fix on a big night out and they're
the perfect foundation for a beautiful dress.
You can also buy control hosiery. I keep well
stocked with good-quality black opaque tights.
My legs are so white I can't bear to get them out, but a great pair
of opaque tights can make them look amazing, especially with
high heels. Steer clear of shiny tights, though, as they're not so flattering.

Over-the-Shoulder Boulder Holders!

Whether you're a big-boobed girl or as flat as a pancake, it's really important to wear the right bra. It's thought that as many as 80 per cent of women wear badly fitting underwear, which is such a shame. What you wear under your clothes can totally change the shape of a dress or shirt and turn it into something special. If you're big, it's vital to get proper support so that you don't put too much pressure on your back. These days you can buy pretty bras, no matter what your size. They can give you more, hoist you up, hold you in, lift and separate. In short, a good bra will make you look young and slim instead of old and droopy.

Buying a bra from a specialist shop is pricey, but I think it's worth splashing out, especially if you need a larger size. I hate to waste money, but if I'm going to invest in one item of clothing it will be a bra. The women who work in these shops are amazing and can tell your size just by looking at you – they don't even need to get their tape measure out.

You can also be measured in most good department stores, but make sure you try the bra for size and ask the assistant for advice. Don't assume you are the same size you've been for years. Age and weight loss or gain usually result in a bra-size change.

DON'T FORGET SHOES AND HANDBAGS

WHAT IS IT WITH WOMEN AND SHOES? SOME HAVE SO MANY PAIRS THEY NEED A SEPARATE CUPBOARD – OR EVEN BEDROOM – FOR THEM! WHEN I'M NOT WORKING, I LIVE IN MY TRAINERS, UGG BOOTS OR SLIPPERS. THAT'S IT. NOT VERY GLAMOROUS, I KNOW, BUT I'VE NEVER BEEN ONE TO OBSESS ABOUT FOOTWEAR.

I must admit, though, that a lovely pair of shoes can do something amazing to an outfit. And I think that if you're going out in the evening wearing a special dress, a pair of killer heels are a must. Just make sure you take some flatties with you in your handbag so you can do a quick swap at the end of the night.

I'm sometimes offered shoes at the end of a photo shoot, so I do have quite a lot, but I'd never pay a fortune if I had to buy them. Honestly, if I'd forked out hundreds of pounds for a pair of, say, Christian Louboutin heels – you know, the posh ones with the red soles – I'd want my money's worth. I'd want to eat, drink and sleep in them, then wear them as slippers, but they're so distinctive you couldn't get away with wearing them all the time. Ray says he'll get a bit of red gloss and paint the bottom of a cheaper pair…no one would know the difference.

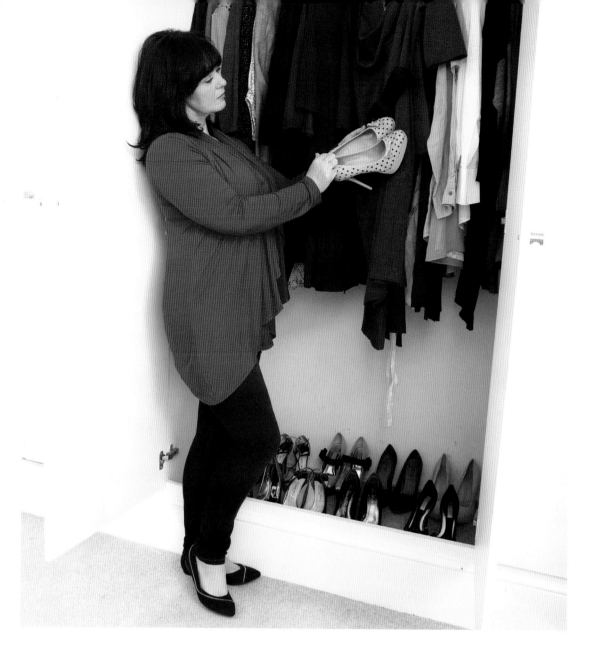

I (almost) never pay a lot for my handbags either. I need great big bags for all the tissues and other rubbish mums have to carry around. I can't understand women who blow a week's wages on a single bag just because it's got a designer label. I have to confess, though, to having a moment of madness recently and spending more than I'd like to admit on a really bling evening bag. It's so sparkly you need sunglasses to look at it, but it is the perfect little bag for a really special night out. I bought it because it is hysterically blingy, though, not because it's got a designer label – in fact, I can't even remember who made it!

STOMACH IN SHOULDERS BACK!

THERE IS NO POINT IN DRESSING WELL IF YOUR POSTURE LETS YOU DOWN. I KNOW THAT I HUNCH MY SHOULDERS FORWARD; IT'S A REACTION TO HAVING BIG BOOBS FROM AN EARLY AGE AND TRYING TO HIDE THEM (I NEEDN'T HAVE BOTHERED REALLY, I DIDN'T FOOL ANYONE).

Just as the right clothes can make you look taller and slimmer, so can a straight back, elegant neck and tucked-in tummy. Stand up straight and you'll look younger and prevent back problems. And the great thing about posture is that it won't cost you a thing.

Even now, because I still feel conscious about my boobs, I have to force myself to sit or stand up straight. If I put my shoulders back and stick my chest out, I feel like I'm saying, 'Just look at these babies!' But I'm determined to practise what I preach and improve my posture in future. I often suffer from a bad back, so it really is something I should do.

Remember, to improve your posture, you need to be conscious of it at all times, not just once a week.

FOLLOW THESE TIPS ON HOW TO
IMPROVE YOUR POSTURE:

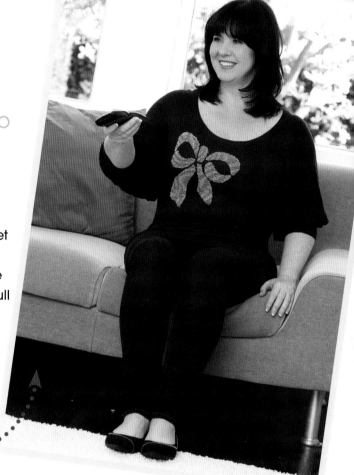

1 Standing up straight with your hands on your hips and your feet a foot apart, tilt your pelvis forward, then back, then find the middle. Relax your shoulders, pull in your tummy and straighten your back.

2 Don't slouch in front of the TV each night. Try to remember to sit with the soles of your feet flat on the floor.

3 Always keep your ears, shoulders and hips in a line. If you remember this rule and regularly correct yourself, you will automatically stand up much straighter.

4 Imagine a string is threaded through the top of your head. Look straight ahead and don't raise or tip your chin. Now pretend someone is gently pulling the string so your neck lengthens. You should find your shoulders relaxing automatically.

5 Keep moving. If you regularly sit at a desk or in front of a computer, there's a good chance you aren't sitting in the correct position. Ask your boss to make sure you have the right equipment and remember to sit up straight, don't let your shoulders droop forward and take breaks every half an hour or so.

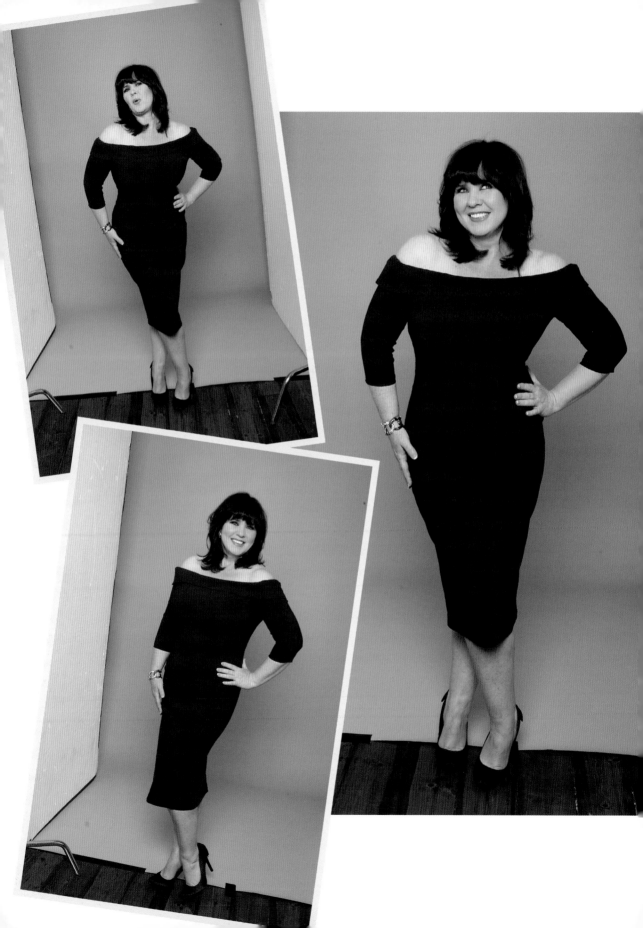

Pretty as a Picture

I've learned from bitter experience that an unflattering photograph can make you feel fat and frumpy. Our own family snaps are bad enough, but these days a photographer can jump out from behind a lamppost and snap me at any time of the day or night. There I'll be with little make-up on, my hair scraped back and a look of panic on my face because I think I'm about to miss the 10.35pm train back home. The results are horrendous!

Usually, however, I know when a picture's about to be taken and have sufficient warning to give it my best shot. I've learned how to stand and what to pull in or push out for the best results. So the next time you see a picture of me in the magazines keep in mind that I'm trying to remember the following rules in order to look my best – it's exhausting!

TRY FOLLOWING THEM YOURSELF AND BE PROUD OF THOSE SNAPS IN THE FAMILY ALBUM:

⟶ *Tighten up a double chin by pressing your tongue against the roof of your mouth just before the picture is taken.*

⟶ *Wear a little more make-up than usual and you won't look so tired – celebrities wouldn't dream of having their photograph taken without a professional make-up artist on hand.*

⟶ *Don't face the camera full on. Stand three-quarters on with one foot in front of the other, so you look your narrowest. And put your hands on your waist or hips.*

⟶ *Remember your posture: push your shoulders back and pull your bum in.*

⟶ *Cross your legs to make them look slimmer.*

⟶ *If you're sitting down, perch on the edge of the chair so your thighs don't spread across the seat.*

⟶ *Believe it or not, there are digital cameras now available that will make you appear 10lb thinner. Honestly! It's not cheating, it's just a little harmless trickery.*

HELP YOURSELF FOR FREE

HAVE YOU EVER DREAMED OF PUTTING YOURSELF IN THE HANDS OF A STYLIST, OR OF WANDERING AROUND A DEPARTMENT STORE WHILE A PERSONAL SHOPPER PICKS OUT A NEW LOOK FOR YOU?

If you have, then perhaps it's time to give yourself a wardrobe workout. Throw out all the clothes you never wear which are cluttering up your cupboards and go shopping for a basic, good-value wardrobe that will make you feel confident, comfortable and attractive.

To do that you don't need to go to the expense of hiring an expert. You can be your own stylist for free. This chapter should have helped you realise what kind of clothes suit your size and shape; now you just have to be tough with yourself and get going. You'll need two spare days to carry out **STEPS ONE** and **TWO** of **THE BIG WARDROBE WORKOUT**. It might feel like a mountain to climb, but it will be worth it. Good luck!

The Big Wardrobe Workout

Step One

The experts reckon that we women only wear 20 per cent of the clothes we own. Empty your wardrobes and drawers of the useless 80 per cent and you'll be able to see what you have and what you still need.

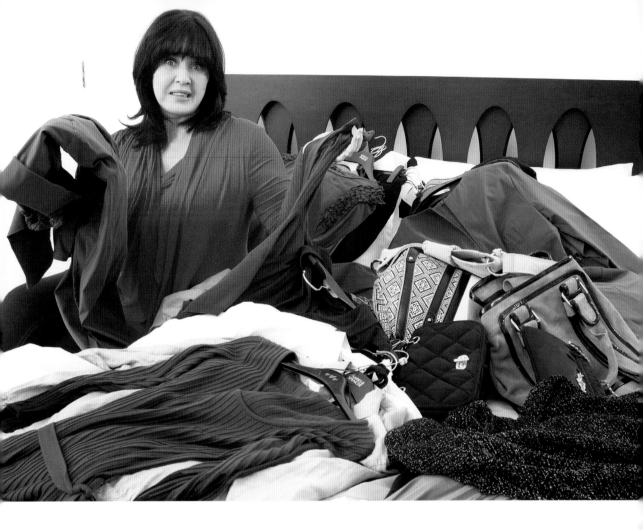

Take out every single item of clothing from your wardrobe and drawers and sort them into four piles: RECYCLE, SELL, MEND AND KEEP.

The RECYCLE pile is for those clothes you never wear, which are fit only for the recycling bin or, better still, the charity shop.

The SELL pile is for clothes that you no longer wear but which could possibly make you some money on an internet auction site or at a car-boot sale.

The MEND pile is for clothes that you never wear because they're missing buttons or need seams repairing.

You should be left with a KEEP pile. This, along with your repaired items of clothing, is the start of your new wardrobe.

Step Two

Now put a second day aside and go shopping – don't worry, it's not going to cost you a penny. Leave the kids behind and wear comfortable shoes, this is going to be hard work. Hit the department and clothing stores and try on the kinds of things you've never thought of wearing before. Be brave. Remember you're not buying today, just storing up knowledge for the future. Take along a notebook and make a list of what suits your shape.

The experts say the perfect wardrobe should be made up of 60 per cent classic items, 20 per cent essential basic items and 20 per cent trendy pieces that will probably date. If you want a checklist of things to buy, then the following items are generally recommended by those in the know: black suit, black heels, trench coat, little black dress, white blouse, cashmere sweater, well-fitted pair of dark jeans, smart skirt, black trousers, boots, blazer-type jacket and assorted T-shirts.

Personally I think it would be a boring world if we all went out dressed in the same capsule wardrobes, but if you're at a loss for ideas – and need to break out of your boring mould – then take the experts' advice and chuck in a few classics of your own.

Now you've done your window shopping you should be left with a list of things to purchase. Try not to shop on impulse – I've made some big mistakes like that. Buying clothes when you need to cheer yourself up always leads to disaster – and often makes you feel even worse as you realise that absolutely *nothing* you try on makes you feel happier/slimmer/younger. Plan ahead, choose your shopping centre carefully and try going when the shops aren't jammed full of people.

When you select an item, think about what's already in your wardrobe and what can be worn with it. Imagine the occasions on which you can wear it and listen to your body – you want clothes that make you feel terrific, confident and comfortable.

If money is a problem, then get organised and open up a separate Wardrobe Fund bank account. Pay in a small amount every month and perhaps ask for contributions for your birthday or Christmas. Promise yourself that the cash in the Wardrobe Fund can only be spent on you, on making you look smart and feel fantastic. It may sound selfish, but there's no reason why you can't keep a tiny share of the family income aside for yourself – if you wait until you have to make a large dent in the weekly budget you'll feel even more guilty!

Alternatively you could get together with your girlfriends to have a clothes swap party. Organised clothes swapping – it's called 'swishing' – is becoming so popular you'll probably be able to find an event being held near you. But why not do your own thing? Provide some nibbles, invite your friends along and tell them to bring a bottle and a bag of clean clothes they no longer wear. You may want to draw up your own rules so that Janice from Number 22 doesn't grab all the best stuff, but usually it's a case of taking only as much as you're prepared to donate. You'll have great fun and hopefully end up with some lovely additions to your wardrobe.

When I absolutely need to buy something new for a big 'do' I can usually never find anything I like. So follow these rules, have a clear-out, do the legwork before the event and take the pressure off. That way the next time you're invited to a posh event, Cinderella will most definitely be ready to go to the ball.

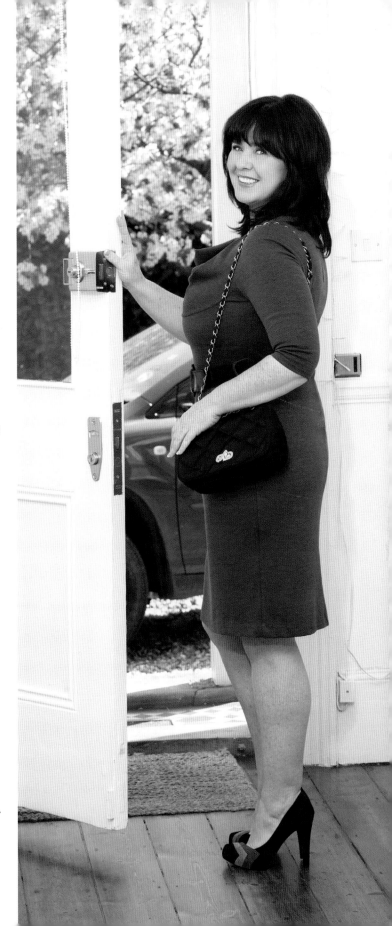

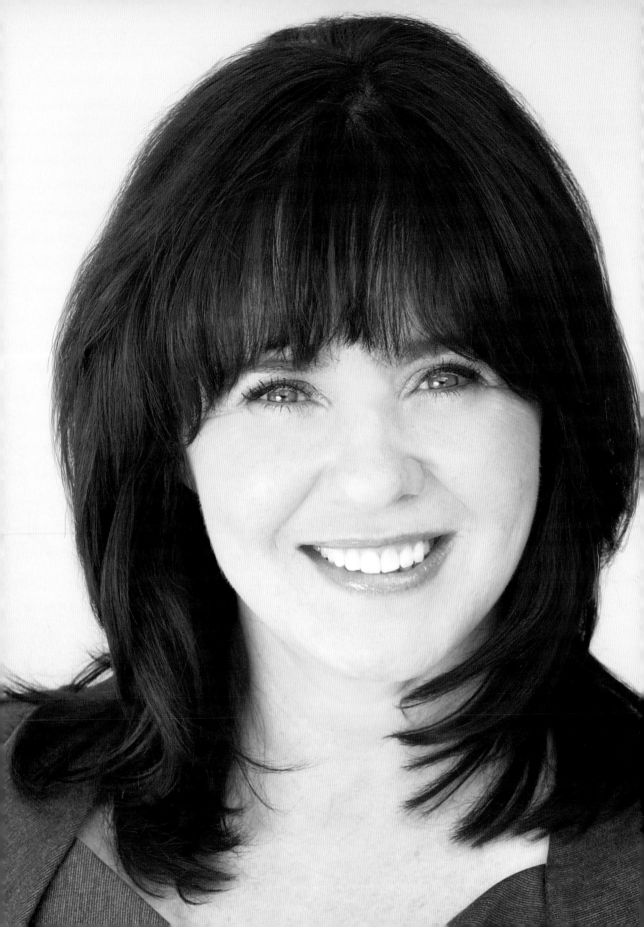

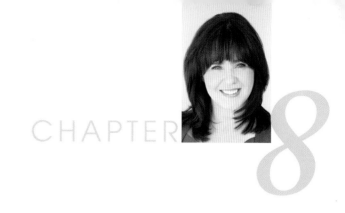

CHAPTER 8

I will survive ...

FEELING
GOOD INSIDE

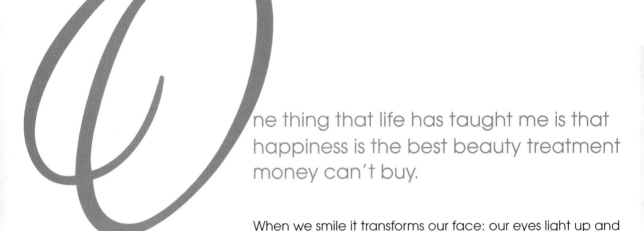

ne thing that life has taught me is that happiness is the best beauty treatment money can't buy.

When we smile it transforms our face: our eyes light up and our worry lines disappear. You must have noticed how a good giggle can make you feel years younger.

The effects of unhappiness and stress can also be physical. When I was miserable and worried about my first marriage, I put on weight, my skin became dull and my hair was lifeless. The allergy problems I had previously suffered from were worse than ever and I was comfort-eating and smoking too much.

If life has bashed you around a bit, there's nothing worse than people telling you to cheer up. You can't easily switch on a smile or suddenly shake yourself out of depression. There may be major things in your life that you need to change and you might even need help from your doctor. But knowing how to de-stress and understanding that a little pampering can lift your spirits is a good first step and might just be enough to break the vicious cycle.

'WHEN WAS THE LAST TIME YOU DEVOTED SOME TIME TO YOURSELF?'

When was the last time you devoted some time to yourself? If the kids are shouting for their tea and there's a huge mountain of ironing to be done, it's difficult to find the time. But by always putting yourself at the bottom of your 'to do' list, happiness can evade you.

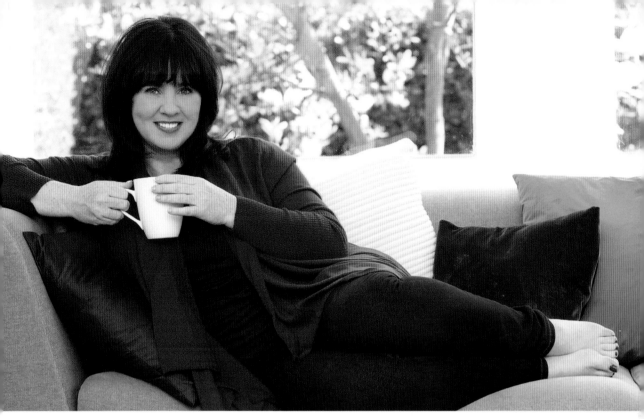

Shiny hair and a new coat of nail varnish are never going to change the world, but they can remind you that you're not ready for the knacker's yard just yet. Take time to care for your appearance, just as we've been talking about throughout this book. Make sure your hair is always clean and in great condition, look after your skin, manicure your nails and paint on a flash of red. I've honestly found that the better I look, the better I feel. And you don't need an expensive wardrobe or spa treatment; just small acts of kindness to yourself will do.

You might also need to start putting yourself ahead of those outside the family. If you're the type who always says yes, even when you want to say no, it's time to work out why you do that. Don't let yourself be intimidated or bullied; stand up for yourself and you'll see how people stop taking you for granted.

In this chapter we'll look at how a good night's sleep and the right food can improve your mood, and I'll be teaching you some magical relaxation techniques I've used in the past when life has got a bit too frantic.

So far we've looked at how to make you shiny and bright on the outside; now it's time to feel good on the inside too.

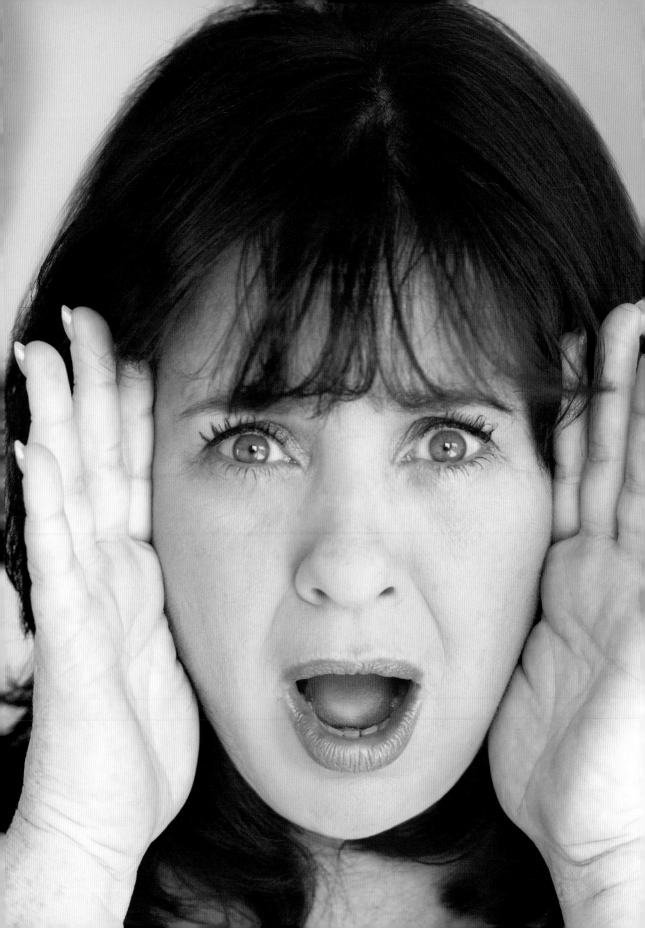

HELP!

SO WHAT IS STRESS? WHY DO WE EXPERIENCE IT, AND WHY DOES IT MAKE US FEEL SO TERRIBLE? STRESS HAS LITTLE TO DO WITH THE AMOUNT OF WORK WE HAVE TO DO – I CAN BE SO BUSY THAT MY FEET DON'T TOUCH THE GROUND, BUT IF I'M DOING SOMETHING I LOVE I STILL FEEL HAPPY.

Not surprisingly I'm at my most relaxed at home and away from the TV studios. The moment I walk through my front door I can feel the weight of the world lifting from my shoulders. On go the slippers, the kettle and the telly – in that order! To be honest, that's when the hard work begins and I become a full-time mum and housewife, but I'm never stressed in my own home.

Real stress is linked to that fight-or-flight reaction that's triggered when we feel frightened, anxious or in danger. This releases hormones that give us extra strength or speed, but these hormones can also stress us out. And if we continue being anxious, then those stress symptoms can make us ill.

Think of a time when you felt overwhelmed by your worries. Were you hit by headaches, tiredness, insomnia, indigestion and skin blemishes? You probably couldn't concentrate, caught coughs and colds easily, overate, drank too much and bit the kids' heads off.

Feeling stressed is bad enough but it's important to learn how to shake it off because, say the experts, continued stress can lead to heart disease, high blood pressure and depression.

Get Counting

Just taking a few moments to breathe deeply can help you feel better. Counting to ten will give you the time to think sensibly about your next move, while the extra oxygen will calm you down and help you relax. The next time someone says something nasty or demands too much of you, just smile and start to count … by the time you reach ten the situation should look much brighter.

Get Tough

I used to be the girl who couldn't say no – *Yes, of course I don't mind having your kids/ driving you to the shops/hosting Christmas/washing your socks* – honestly I was pathetic. But when I married Ray he made me stick up for myself. I can be very easily intimidated and he made me realise it was OK to refuse requests. He made me stand up to my first husband, Shane, my huge family and everyone else who wanted something from me. Not in a horrible way, just so that I could put myself first without feeling guilty. Now I realise I've wasted too many years worrying about what others think – stuff 'em!

Get Organised

You can't change the number of hours in the day, but you can decide what you do with them. Prioritise the jobs that are most important and think about binning the rest. Or set your alarm to get you up fifteen minutes earlier every day and make good use of that time, even if it's just to give yourself fifteen minutes' peace for a morning cup of tea before the madness begins. You should also ask for help and delegate jobs to other members of the family – draw up a rota to share out the housework a bit. Grit your teeth and tackle those jobs you've been putting off – fifteen minutes a day spent on getting the house in order will make you feel better in the long run. You could also begin filling in the family diary and booking in events to look forward to: a Saturday picnic with friends, a night in with the girls or having another family over for Sunday lunch.

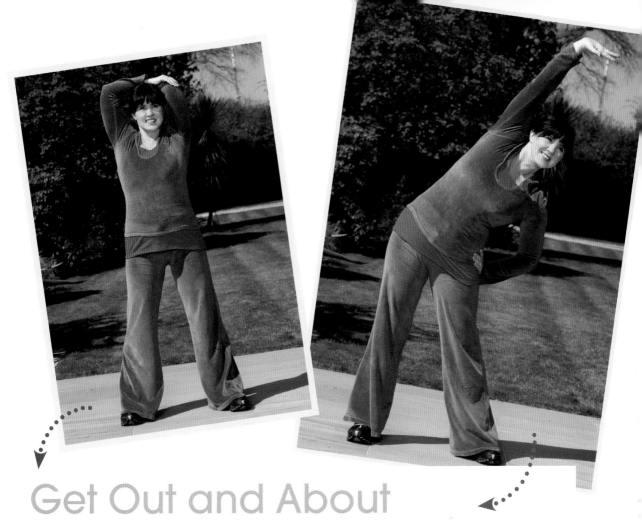

Get Out and About

It's not easy motivating yourself when you're feeling low, but I promise that even a short walk will make you feel much better. Exercise will give you extra energy, more self-confidence and some precious time to yourself. If you're really not into sport, why not try a new hobby? Amateur dramatics or night-school classes are a great way to make new friends. Or you could offer to be a volunteer at your local school, hospital or dogs' home – whatever you find rewarding and fulfilling.

Get to Bed

Sleeping on a problem is always a good idea, but it can be easier said than done. Stress can stop us sleeping and lack of sleep can make us stressed – it's a disaster! A regular sleep pattern is really important, so try to get a solid eight hours to set you up for the following day. If you're having problems sleeping, look out for my tips on this later in the chapter.

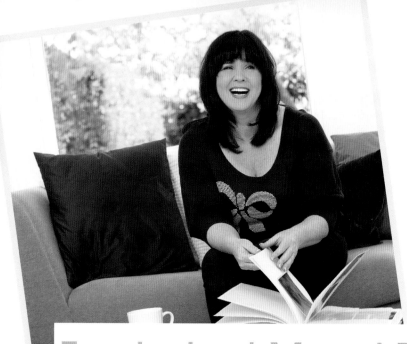

'A PHOTO
ALBUM WILL LIFT
YOUR SPIRITS
EVERY TIME
YOU OPEN IT'

Ten Instant Mood Boosters

- *Make a CD of your favourite songs*

Keep copies in the car or in your handbag. There are songs that remind me of my wedding to Ray, of when the kids were little, of my parents, my sisters and friends, and each one makes me smile as soon as I hear it.

- *Do something nice for somebody else*

Thinking of others occasionally won't turn you into a doormat. Write a letter to a friend, do some shopping for an elderly neighbour or help a stranger struggling with a pushchair. It's amazing how good these things make you feel.

- *Sort out a cupboard*

You know the cupboard I mean: the one full of junk that's now getting seriously out of hand. Get a bin liner and chuck out those useless receipts, the lifetime collection of plastic bags and the stack of empty margarine tubs. Feeling better already?

- *Have a stretch*

If you're feeling unhappy, the chances are your body is tense too. Give each part of your body a good stretch, starting at your toes and finishing with your face muscles. Tense and stretch each muscle, then relax – this is good first thing in the morning and last thing at night.

• Enjoy a deep, warm bubble bath

Flick back to Chapter 3 to see how to set up your own home spa. A long soak in a deliciously scented bath is always a great pick-me-up.

• Think naughty thoughts

Every so often I have a very fruity dream about my skating hero and heart-throb Christopher Dean. It's marvellous. I never go so far as breaking my vows to Ray, but I wake up with a smile on my face! If you're feeling low, try conjuring up your favourite sexual fantasy – so long as it's only in your head, who's to know?

• Make a family photo album

I used to keep all my pictures in boxes, and once the lids were on they never saw the light of day. When I began putting them in albums, it gave me such pleasure to go through old photographs from my childhood and pictures of the kids growing up. These days it's tempting to leave digital snaps in the camera or on a computer – print them out and get them in an album that will lift your spirits every time you open it.

• Escape into a gripping novel

I spend too many hours on trains travelling between our house in Cheshire and work in London, but at least I can spend the time with my nose in a good book. I can easily lose myself in a bit of chick lit, and the stories give me another universe to live in when this one gets a bit tough!

• Use relaxation techniques to drift off

Meditation sounds very far out and hippy-ish but it's just a way of finding peace and quiet and improving your mood. Choose a moment when you have the house to yourself and grab some 'me' time. I'll explain the technique I use at the end of this chapter.

• Boogie your blues away!

I dance around the house to keep fit and keep my weight down, but dancing is also a great way to instantly boost your mood, especially if you jig along to a favourite song. Exercise releases feel-good chemicals that will make you smile quicker than you can say, 'I'm in the mood…'

Eat Yourself Happy

I'm never happier than when in front of a large plate of pasta, in the certain knowledge that there's a lovely chocolate pudding waiting for me. What's not to smile about? But after the initial gluttony, the guilt kicks in and happiness can turn into gloom.

I can't imagine a life without these favourite things, but the secret is to have a little of what you fancy while remaining in control. Alcohol, biscuits and chocolate can be as good a pick-me-up as a facial, but the trick is not to have the entire bottle, packet or bar.

The experts will tell you that sugary carbohydrates such as cakes, biscuits and bread are bottom of the list when it comes to mood-boosting foods, but that's not to say you can't enjoy the occasional treat. On a day-to-day basis, though, think about replacing white bread with wholemeal or swapping that HobNob for a health bar. Boring, I know, but if you are feeling low, it's worth considering.

HERE ARE SOME OTHER HAPPY MEALS:

- Oily fish, such as salmon or tuna, is full of **OMEGA 3**, which is a great brain food and is said to lift your mood.

- Leafy green vegetables are rich in **VITAMIN B** and will have a positive effect on your nervous system. Spinach is especially high in minerals believed to fight anxiety and depression.

- Walnuts are high in **OMEGA 3**, while Brazil nuts contain the natural mood booster **SELENIUM**.

- Chocolate, particularly the dark variety, is said to stimulate natural antidepressants in the brain.

- The smell of lemons has been proven to make people feel happier – why not try slicing one into a jug of iced water, or putting a few drops of lemon essential oil in an oil burner to fragrance your bedroom or living room?

- **PROTEIN-RICH FOODS**, such as lean meat, eggs, yoghurt, fish, soya beans and tofu, will give you more energy and therefore lift your mood.

- Hot chilli peppers contain chemicals that release **ENDORPHINS** and make you feel happier. Chillis can also increase blood flow and heart rate, so they stimulate nerve endings and get you in the mood for love. That should cheer you up!

- Go bananas for bananas, the fruit that makes you feel cheerful. It's down to a chemical called **TRYPTOPHAN**, a type of protein that the body converts into a feel-good hormone called **SEROTONIN**. Bananas are also high in carbs, so they'll give you an energy boost, too.

- A balanced breakfast is important to give you a great start to the day. Mix good carbs such as fruit or wholemeal toast with a protein food like eggs or yoghurt and you should avoid the drops in energy that lead to mood swings. Remember to eat lots of little snacks through the day rather than three big meals – another way to avoid mood swings.

- Drinking tea, coffee and alcohol in huge quantities isn't a great idea because the caffeine in the tea and coffee can ruin your sleep patterns while alcohol is a depressant. If caffeine keeps you awake, avoid tea and coffee after 2pm. A glass of wine may help you sleep, but you shouldn't be drinking more than two units a day, which is roughly equivalent to one small glass.

- Dehydration will make you feel tired and moody, so make sure you drink plenty of water. This doesn't come naturally to me – I never really feel thirsty – but I'm trying to train myself to get my eight glasses a day!

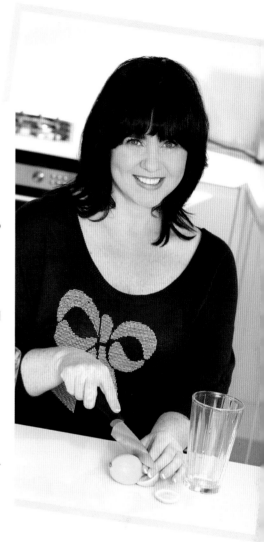

'THE SMELL OF LEMONS HAS BEEN PROVEN TO MAKE PEOPLE FEEL HAPPIER'

Grin and Bear it

Introducing exercise into your daily routine will make you feel better inside as well as out. But did you know there are exercises that can also perk up the tired bits of your face? Aerobics for that double chin! You might want to try these manoeuvres in privacy because, effective though they may be, pretty they ain't! Do them daily and you really will feel the difference.

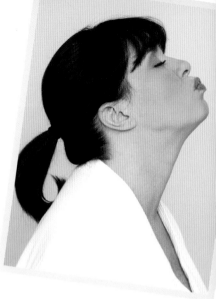

- *Jaw-Line Workout*
Sit upright, tilt your head back and look at the ceiling, keep your mouth closed and begin a chewing movement. **REPEAT TWENTY TIMES**

- *Double-Chin Workout*
Jut out your chin and tip it up slightly so that your neck feels comfortably stretched. Push your lower lip out and over your top lip. Now push the tip of your tongue against the roof of your mouth behind your teeth. Keep increasing the pressure and hold for five seconds. Relax, then repeat the exercise, this time holding the position for ten seconds. Relax and repeat again, this time holding for fifteen seconds or for as long as you can.

- *Cheeky Workout*
Smile as widely as you can into a mirror. Keep your lips closed and the corners of your mouth turned up. Wrinkle your nose and see your cheek muscles move upwards. **REPEAT FIVE TIMES.**

- *Eye Workout*
Press two fingers against either side of your head, next to your eyes. Wake up the muscles there by opening and closing your eyes quickly fifteen times. Relax. **REPEAT FIVE TIMES**

- *Forehead Workout*
Sit up straight, bring your eyebrows down as far as you can, wrinkle your nose and flare your nostrils – I told you to do this in private! Hold for ten seconds, then relax. **REPEAT TEN TIMES.**

Relight My Fire...

Going on tour with The Nolans last year was the best thing I've done in a long, long while. I loved being able to perform again, and the fans seemed to love having us back. I had my entire family with me – Shane Junior and Jake were supporting us, while Ciara packed her schoolwork and did her lessons on the tour bus. Ray came too, and of course I had my sisters right alongside me. If any experience was designed to make you feel good, then that was it.

I'm not suggesting you pack your dance shoes and sparkly dresses and head off on a tour around Britain's theatres, but rediscovering something you love is a great idea. Perhaps you and your partner used to trip the light fantastic every Saturday night but have given all that up for a snooze on the sofa followed by **Match of the Day***. Or maybe you were a regular at the local cinema but these days find yourself not knowing what the big films are from one year to the next. Your greatest pleasure may have been simply walking in the park, but now a trip to the shops is all you can be bothered with.*

Why not rekindle an old passion or even find a new one?
Here are TEN EXPERIENCES *I want you to tick off in the next six months:*

➡ *Have a candlelit dinner.*
➡ *Dance until you're breathless.*
➡ *Learn a new skill.*
➡ *Climb the highest hill in your area.*
➡ *Have sex somewhere other than in bed.*
➡ *Buy tickets for a concert.*
➡ *Swim in the sea.*
➡ *Beat your kids or grandkids at a computer game.*
➡ *Stroke more than five different animal species.*
➡ *Visit a fairground and ride a rollercoaster.*

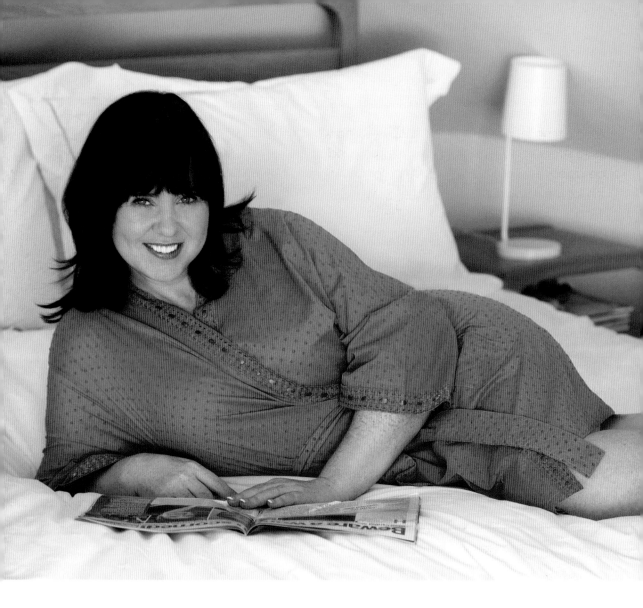

BEAUTY SLEEP

I'M KNOWN AS RIP VAN WINKLE IN MY FAMILY BECAUSE I CAN DOZE OFF ANYWHERE. WHEN WE GO ON HOLIDAY I'M ASLEEP BEFORE THE PLANE TAKES OFF AND I DON'T WAKE UP UNTIL IT'S LANDED AGAIN. RAY SAYS I'M THE WORST CAR PASSENGER IN THE WORLD BECAUSE I DOZE OFF BEFORE WE'VE EVEN LEFT OUR DRIVEWAY.

The only time in my life I had trouble sleeping was during my stint on *Dancing on Ice*. I was so stressed out I used to toss and turn and scream and shout out in my sleep. My face aged ten years overnight, so I know how important it is to get your beauty sleep, both for the way you look and the way you feel inside.

If you have problems sleeping, make sure you don't have too much to eat or drink before bedtime; as I said earlier, you should avoid tea or coffee after 2pm and only have a light snack before bed. It's also a good idea to avoid working on the computer before bedtime, and don't watch telly in bed. You don't want to be all puffed out through exercise before you go to sleep either; the only breathlessness you should experience is the type that comes from getting frisky with your partner (this will help you sleep and is the exception to the rule).

One tried and trusted way to promote a good night's sleep is to have a soak in a warm relaxing bath before bedtime, and it's also important to make sure your bedroom isn't too hot or cold.

If you tend to lie awake worrying about jobs that need doing, put a notebook and pencil on your bedside table and jot down thoughts as they occur to you to get those worries out of your head and onto the paper.

Perhaps you're not sleeping because of noise or too much light in the bedroom? In which case, try ear plugs or an eye mask.

Try going to bed at the same time every night; the experts say a regular routine is important for a good night's sleep. You could listen to soft music while you drift off or ask your partner for a relaxing massage...wherever that leads!

I've heard that some people count backwards in order to drift off, starting at 1,000 and counting down as far as they need to. Alternatively, imagine you're in a favourite place – your garden or a beach perhaps. You can feel the warmth of the sun on your face and body and smell the scent of the flowers or the salt of the sea. Gently breathe in and out and feel your chest relaxing. Lie still with your eyes closed and relax until you drop off. Imagine the same place and sensations whenever you have difficulty sleeping and it should become easier to relax each time.

HELP YOURSELF FOR FREE

IT'S REALLY DIFFICULT TO FIND TIME FOR YOURSELF, I KNOW. IT SEEMS LIKE EVERYONE WANTS A PIECE OF YOU AND I OFTEN FIND MYSELF TORN BETWEEN WORK, FAMILY AND FRIENDS.

The relaxation techniques below are fantastic when you need a little calm in your life. They slow things down in an instant, lower your blood pressure and heart rate and ease tension in the body. Adapt them to suit your needs and use them whenever the chaos gets too much.

And Relax

1 Switch off your phone, the television, the radio and tell yourself to ignore any outside noises (it's not always possible to have an empty house, so learn how to shut out distractions).

2 Make yourself comfortable, either sitting or lying down. Softly close your eyes and breathe in a regular rhythm – in through your nose and out through your mouth.

3 Tense each part of your body, starting at your feet. Scrunch your toes for a few seconds, then relax them. Next flex your feet at the ankles, hold for a few seconds, then relax. Tense your calves, hold for a few seconds, then relax. Do this for each part of the body, travelling through your legs, bottom, stomach, chest, shoulders, elbows, wrists and fingers. When you get to your head, scrunch your facial muscles tightly, hold for a few seconds, then relax. Finish by raising your eyebrows for a few seconds, then letting them fall.

4 Stay still for a few minutes more, letting any thoughts drift from your head. Continue to breathe deeply, in through the nose, out through the mouth.

5 When you are absolutely calm, open your eyes and slowly sit up.

And Relax Some More

1 Lie on the floor or your bed, close your eyes and relax. Softly breathe in and out, in through the nose and out through the mouth.

2 Imagine your body is so heavy it begins to sink through the floor or mattress. Your feet are so heavy they start to sink lower than the rest of your body, then your legs, your bottom, your stomach and chest. Feel your arms become heavy and sink downwards, then your shoulders and finally your head. Feel your eyes and cheeks and mouth and jaw sink into the floor or mattress.

3 Your entire body is getting heavier and heavier and you sink further and further down into the floor or mattress.

4 Let go of all your cares and worries and stay like that for as long as you want, breathing deeply.

5 When you are absolutely relaxed, open your eyes and slowly sit up.

Stroke Your Cares Away

You only need a few moments to do this soothing temple massage. I find it calms me down and somehow gives me more energy all at the same time.

1 Sit up straight, close your eyes and begin to breathe deeply, in through the nose, out through the mouth.

2 Place the tips of three fingers flat against either temple and be aware of the gentle pulse of the blood in your veins.

3 As you breathe out, press your fingertips against your head, hold for seven seconds, then relax. Repeat five times, each time on an outward breath.

4 Cover your face with both hands and take seven deep breaths in and out.

5 Lower your hands and take three more deep breaths before opening your eyes.

Soak Your Cares Away

If you can keep the rest of the family out of the bathroom for long enough, a leisurely soak in a warm bath is a great stress reliever. Light some candles, play your favourite music and sip a naughty glass of wine or cold soft drink. These ingredients from your kitchen and garden will help make the experience even more relaxing.

Vanilla
Sprinkle a few drops of vanilla essence into the water and be calmed by the sweet, soothing, delicious smell.

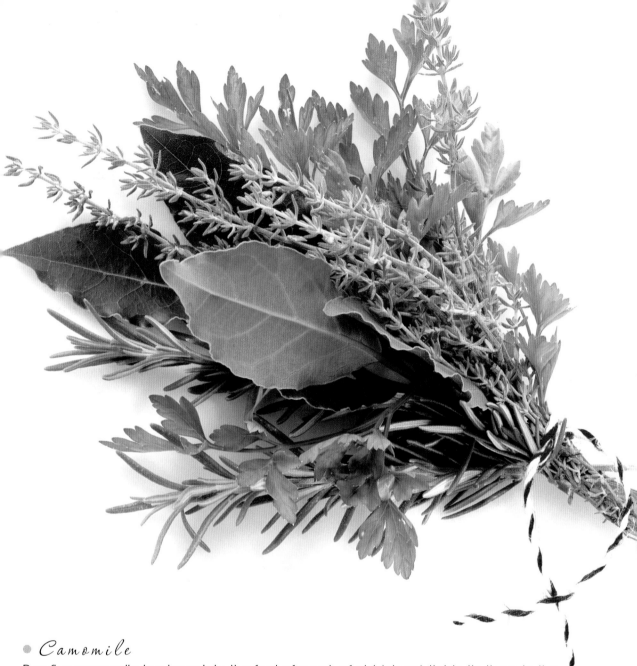

● *Camomile*

Pop five camomile tea bags into the foot of a pair of old (clean) tights, tie them to the taps and let hot water run through them as your bath fills. Float a few wafter-thin orange slices on the surface for a relaxing, yet energising bath.

● *Herbs*

Place any fresh herbs, for example rosemary, lavender or mint (get them from the garden if you can) in your tights bath bag. Tie the bag to the taps and let the hot water run through it. Really relaxing.

IN THE
MOOD YET?

WHEN I LOOK BACK THROUGH THIS BOOK I'M AMAZED AT HOW MANY TIPS AND TRICKS I'VE PICKED UP OVER THE YEARS.

I've loved jotting down all the advice I've been given and I hope each page will help you look and feel a million dollars. But I'll let you into a secret: every section is a great reminder of what I should be doing, because I don't always take my own advice!

Remember how I said I used to sit in the house, dressed in tracksuit bottoms, eating biscuits and feeling fat and fed up? Well, I still sometimes sit in the house dressed in tracksuit bottoms. I still eat biscuits – just not the whole packet – and I quite often feel fed up. I've just learned how to do something about it.

I've also learned how to be honest with myself, about which clothes suit me and when to say no to people. I now know who I am: a mum of three in her mid-forties with a loving husband, great friends and family and a wonderful, if demanding, job. I look in the mirror and think, Not bad. Not perfect, but not bad…considering.

I've been through unhappy times, unhealthy times and times of huge doubt and insecurity, and I find it amazing that it's taken me until now to feel this good. We only have one life and we owe it to ourselves to make it the best it can be. Some might say it's shallow to worry too much about looks and beauty, but I'm living proof that by looking better on the outside, you feel better on the inside, too.

My life has changed so much since I lost some weight, got fitter and started looking after myself. Now I feel more confident and I'm determined not to go back to my bad old ways. Just the other day I worked out that I'd spent far too many hours standing on our bathroom scales, so I chucked them in the bin. Over the years I've yo-yo dieted from a size 22 at my heaviest to a size 8 at my tiniest, and I want to live the rest of my life not stressing about pounds, stones and size tags. I've made a vow to myself to be healthier and happier, and so far that appears to go hand in hand with a body I'm content with.

I'll never again have the figure of that teenage girl who first stepped onto the stage to sing with her sisters, but going back on tour with them showed me I could still get on stage and sing and dance for two hours without collapsing with exhaustion.

I've come this far by not putting myself last all the time. Yes, I have a great supporter in my husband, Ray, and loads of love from the rest of my family, but it's only by looking after myself that I've reached this point in my life. I hope this book inspires you to find that place, too.

I know it's a cliché, but real beauty does come from within. You can be the most beautiful woman in the world, but if you're a wicked person, a poor friend or a selfish so-and-so, you will never be attractive to other people. In my work you get to meet the most extraordinarily attractive people, but if they're stuck-up or self-centred, their beauty seems to vanish into thin air. And believe me, I've met quite a few like that!

I think we should all remember to cherish those we love and be kind to complete strangers. But most importantly we should give ourselves a break. It's one thing to know how to get shiny hair, manicured nails and beautiful skin; it's another to give yourself a hard time if you don't always look your best. Life isn't a competition after all.

So still have your chocolate biscuit and pyjama days, still pull on your tracksuit when you feel like it. Just remember that when you want to, you can go out there and knock 'em dead.

Good luck and lots of love,

Coleen xx

INDEX

A

accessories 117, 188
alcohol 40, 163, 211

B

bathing and showers 71–2, 73, 74–5, 77, 86–9, 209, 215, 218–19
bedding 105
bikini line 78, 79, 80–1
blusher 59
body shape 20–1, 179, 181, 182
bras 181
breathing 206
bronzer 60, 83
brows 44–5
bunions 137

C

caffeine 211
celebrity beauty 68–9
cellulite 76–7
cleansing 17, 32–3, 63, 71, 134, 137
    see also bathing and showers
clothes 174–5, 176
    apple body shape 181
    athletic body shape 182
    for big and small boobs 183–4
    colours 188
    dressing to slim 186, 188
    dressing your age 178
    hourglass body shape 181
    to lengthen legs 183
    pear body shape 179
    shoes and handbags 138, 190–1
    swapping 199
    underwear 188–9
    wardrobe workout 196–9

coffee 40, 211, 215
collagen 37, 43
concealers 53
conditioner 100–1, 102, 118, 120–1
confidence 23, 69, 206
cosmetics
    see make-up

D

dancing 149, 150, 209, 213
dandruff 25, 102–3
dehydration 211
depilatory creams 80
depression 202, 208–9, 213
diet 17, 23, 24, 40, 44, 102
    alcohol 163
    cellulite 77
    hair and nails 102, 104–5, 133
    mind set 158
    mood enhancing 210–11
    motivators 164–5
    sample menus 160–1
    weight loss 26
    see also vitamins and minerals
dyeing hair 94, 110–11, 113

E

electrolysis 80
epilators 79
exercise 23, 26–7, 76, 140–1, 146, 148, 151, 156, 166, 207, 215
    bottom 170
    cycling 154
    dancing 147, 150
    domestic chores 152
    facial muscles 212
    ice skating 154–5

sex 157
swimming 154
thighs 171
tummy and sides 168–9
upper arms 167
walking 152
    see also diet
exfoliating 35, 63, 70–1, 72, 79, 86, 88, 134, 141, 143
extensions 116–17
eyes 44–5, 54–7, 60, 64, 212

F

face
    exercises 212
    masks 62
    shapes 16, 18–19, 106–7
    skin types 16–17
    see also make-up
fake tan 82–3
false eyelashes 57
false nails 126, 132–3
fashion
    see clothes
feet 124–5, 134, 136–9, 140–3
food
    see diet
foundation 52–3, 58

H

hair 37, 92–3
    accessories 117
    blow-drying 114–15
    cleansing 96–101
    colours 94, 110–11, 113
    dandruff 102–3
    and diet 102, 104–5
    extensions 116–17

hairdressers 94, 109
removal 44–5, 78–81
split ends 103
styles 18, 19, 24, 94, 106–7
thinning 102
treatments 118, 120–1
types 24–5, 96–7
hands 124–7, 129, 130–1, 140,
141–3
hobbies 207, 213
    see also exercise

I
ice skating 154

L
laser hair removal 80, 81
lips 45, 58, 60, 64

M
make-up 17, 18, 48–9
    blusher 59, 60
    bronzer 60
    brushes etc 50
    cheeks 59
    eyes 54–7
    foundation 52–3, 60
    hints and tips 60
    lips 58, 60
    removal 33
    self-tanning 82–3
manicures 125, 130–1
mascara 55, 56–7
masks 62, 143
massage 76, 102, 133, 136, 139,
143, 215, 218
moisturising 45
    body 72–3, 76

face 17, 34, 60
hands and feet 129, 134, 136,
    137, 141, 142, 143

N
nails 37, 105, 126, 130–3, 134, 136,
137, 141

P
pedicures 125, 134, 136
perfume 84–5
photographs 195, 209
pilates 151
posture 151, 192–3, 195
powder (make-up) 53

R
relaxation techniques 27, 208,
209, 215, 216–19

S
scrubs
    see exfoliating
self-image 68–9
sex 157, 209, 213
shampoo 98, 100, 102–3, 133
shaving 78–9
shoes 138, 190
skin 30–1, 69, 105
    aging 36–7, 40, 124–7
    care products 37, 62–4
    diet 40, 43
    dry brushing body 70–1
    steaming 35
    types 16–17
    see also bathing and
    showers; cleansing;
    exfoliating; moisturising;

sun protection
sleep 44, 157, 207, 211,
214–15
smoking 39
split ends 103
spots 17, 30, 33
steaming 35
stress 27, 157, 202, 205 206,
208–9, 213
    see also relaxation
    techniques
sun protection 34, 37, 52,
82–3, 129
surgery 39
swimming 154

T
tanning 82–3
tea 211, 215
teeth 47, 64
toner 33, 64

U
underwear 188–9
V
vitamins and minerals 37,
40, 43, 105, 133, 210

W
water 40, 44, 163, 211
waxing 80
weight management
    see diet; exercise
wrinkles 30–1, 33, 34, 36–7,
43, 64
    see also make-up;
    skin

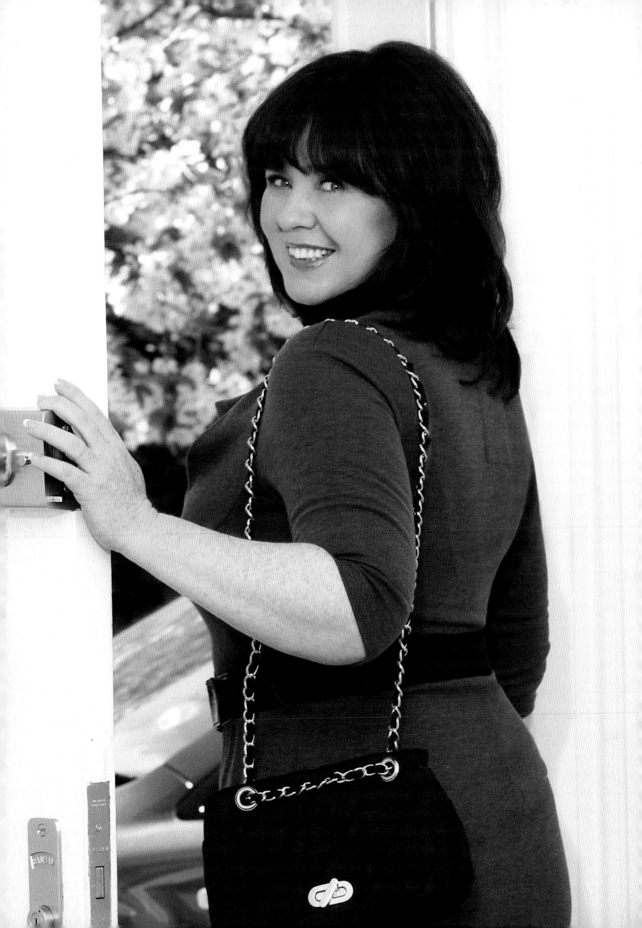